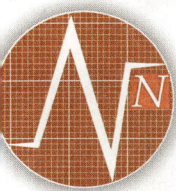

Nursing Next Live

ONE NATION / ONE e-RESOURCE

The Next Level of **NURSING EDUCATION**

WHY CHOOSE NURSING NEXT LIVE?

- ✓ First Digital Learning platform for All Nursing Competitive & Undergraduate Exams with Futuristic Approach
- ✓ We are bringing Learning to People, Instead of People going for learning!
- ✓ Concept-Based Teaching by TOP Medical & Nursing Educators (The Masterminds)
- ✓ "Quality Content" & "Smart-Study" Approach
- ✓ One-in-All, All-in-One! Nothing Beyond
- ✓ 360 Degree Approach for your complete Preparation
- ✓ Most Up-to-date Content
- ✓ Monthly National Scholarship and Mega Assessment Tests
- ✓ Best Guidance & Support at every step
- ✓ Best Interface with Unique & Advance Features
- ✓ Buy CBS Nursing Books at Special Discounts/ Cashbacks

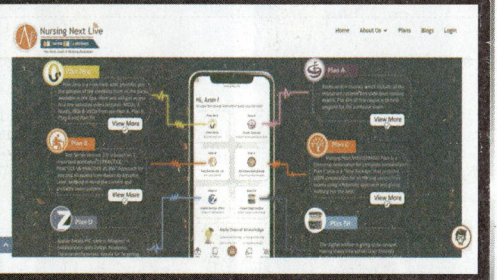

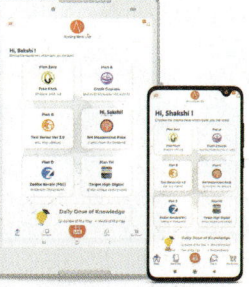

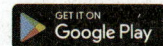
GET IT ON Google Play

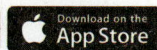
Download on the App Store

Coming Soon

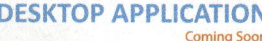
DESKTOP APPLICATION
Coming Soon

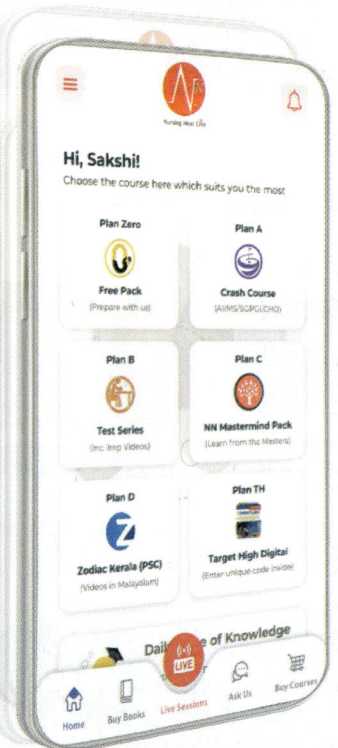

The Complete Package

- 40,000+ MCQs with Rationale
- 2000+ Hours of Recorded video lectures (Covering All Subjects/All Topics /Imp Topics Chanting Videos/Exam Discussions/LMR/IBQ & VBQs Discussions)
- 150+ Previous years' question papers covering all National & State Level Exams (2020-10)
- Monthly Live Doubt Sessions
- 200+ Newly Created Subject-wise cum Topic-wise Test, Mini Test & Grand Tests based on all important National Exams like AIIMS, PGIMER, JIPMER, DSSSB, RRB & ESIC, also State level exams like Kerala PSC
- 1500+ E-Notes/Flash cards of all the subjects for Last-Minute Revision
- 1000+ Image-based Questions with Rationale
- 200+ Video-based Questions with Rationale
- Monthly National Scholarship Test with Reward points
- 200+ CBS Nursing Books available for purchase

60K USERS 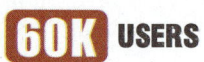 **1000+** CITIES Covered 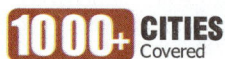 **60+** Mins Daily Average Time of users 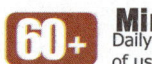 **4.7** RATINGS Google Play Store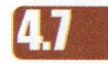

TOP SELECTIONS
AIIMS NORCET 2020
(What Students Say About Nursing Next Live)

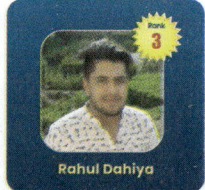
Rank 3
Rahul Dahiya

Rank 12
Nisha Singla

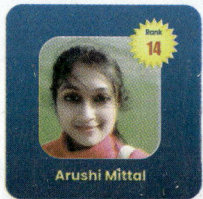
Rank 14
Arushi Mittal

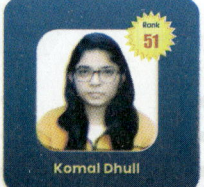
Rank 51
Komal Dhull

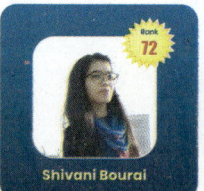
Rank 72
Shivani Bourai

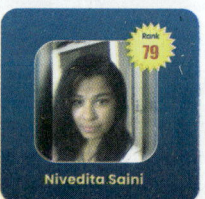
Rank 79
Nivedita Saini

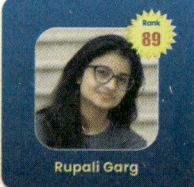
Rank 89
Rupali Garg

What's New?

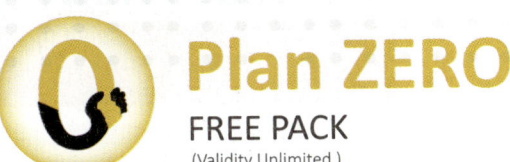

Plan ZERO
FREE PACK
(Validity Unlimited)

Nothing comes first to us than providing you the right direction to your preparation and helping you to succeed. Plan Zero is a Free Pack that provides you the glimpses of the contents from all the packs available in the app. Here you will get access to a few selective video lectures, MCQs, E Notes, IBQs & VBQs from our Plan A, Plan B, Plan C, and Plan TH. This pack will help you to get an overview of the content of all the courses and also equip you with the smart study pattern approach.

Aim:
- Glimpses of complete content in a systemic manner
- Covering Basics of Everything in the form of Subject-wise MCQs, Grand Tests, Videos, E-Notes, IBQs & VBQs, Previous Year Papers and lots more

Best for:
- Students who are going to start their preparation and want to know how Nursing Next Live can help them in their success.
- Students who are completely prepared for their exams and want to give the final touch to their preparation

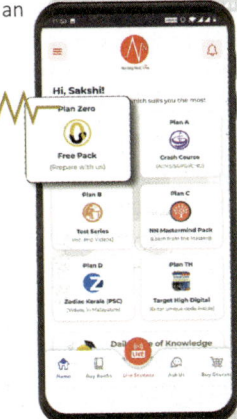

What all you will get

- **2000+** MCQs with Rationale covering All Subjects, Important Topics
- **150+** E-Notes covering All Subjects, Selective important Topics
- **100+** Hours of Lectures covering All Subjects (Topic-wise/Imp Topics/Chanting/Exam Discussions)
- **100+** IBQs & VBQs of All Subjects
- **15** Most Recent/Previous Years Papers with Rationale
- **5+** Grand Test & Bonus Test based on Real Time Exam Pattern
- Daily Dose of Knowledge— Word of the Day, Fact of the Day, Practice Pearls, Question of the Day
- Unsolved & Solved Question Papers of BSc 1st to 4th Year in a consolidated manner covering all Important Universities (Forthcoming)
- Monthly National Scholarship Test with Special Descount for Top Rankers
- How to Prepare for Exams (in the form of Study Planner/Videos)
- Complete Access to Target High Extra Edge Section – which includes additional MCQs & Golden Points in Video Form

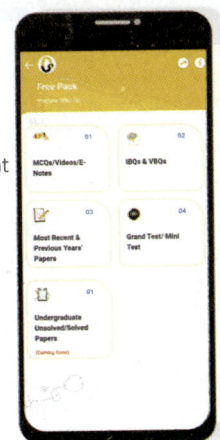

Special Features

| Study Plans | Success Stories | Daily Dose of Knowledge | Blogs | National Scholarship Test (NST) | Any Doubt Ask Us | Exam Notification | Buy CBS Books | Bookmark | Download Videos |

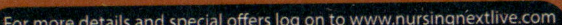

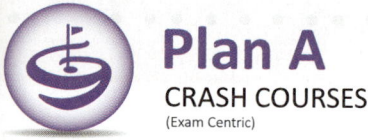

Plan A
CRASH COURSES
(Exam Centric)

Exam-centric courses which include all the important national and state level nursing exams. The aim of this course is to help students prepare for a particular exam. We have come out with AIIMS NORCET 2020, SGPGI, CHO & Target Kerala PSC Crash Courses and this will keep adding on as and when any exam notification announces. All Crash Courses cover the complete syllabus and are based on the real-time pattern of the particular exams.

All crash courses are having detailed content in the form of Subject-wise/Topic-wise Qs with Rationale, a variety of Grand Tests based on Real-Time Pattern, E-Notes for LMR & Chanting/Imp Topics Videos by the TOP Educators. All our Crash Courses are highly reasonable in Price and are value for money.

Aim:
• To polish your knowledge with Live Test & Videos on daily basis
• To focus on Quality instead of Quantity. To give you only the Best learning experience
• Providing you most personalized and customized study material that suits all your preparation needs

Best for:
• The students who are targeting any particular exam
• Working Professionals who have a limited time to study can prepare well from this pack in a less period of time.
• The students who have prepared well for the exam, but want to gain a last-minute momentum
• Students who have just started their preparation, but do not know what to study, or from where to start

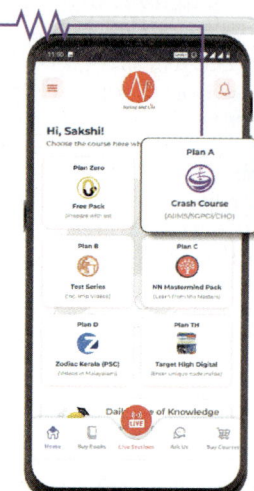

What all you will get

Plan A1 – CHO Crash Course (Validity 60 Days)
• **35+** Subject-wise Tests & Grand Tests (including Bonus Tests & Previous Years Papers)
• **1500+** Questions with rationale
• **70+** E-notes for last-minute revision covering all the important topics as per the syllabus of CHO
• **30+** (Duration of 30+ Hours) Pre-recorded Videos given by top faculties in Hinglish covering every important topic from exam point of view

Plan A2 – AIIMS NORCET 2020 Crash Course (Validity 90 Days)
• **60+** Live Tests Subject-wise based on AIIMS Delhi pattern
• **1500+** Qs with Rationale including MCQs, IBQs, VBQs, Clinical skills, Priority setting, and case study
• **15+** Mock Test, Revision Test, and Grand Tests based on Real-time pattern of AIIMS Delhi with Negative Marking and National Level Ranking
• All Subject-wise Tests & Grand Tests are with Detailed Rationale
• **140+** Last-Minute Revision Notes based on Frequently asked Topics of previous Years
• **12+** Videos on Chanting Session by Top Educators/Subject Experts
• **35+** Multiple videos on special tricks for non-nursing subjects, tips on memory retention, strategies to attempt exams, etc.
• Success Guaranteed as we have had 150+ Selections (Rank 3 to 5k) in AIIMS NORCET 2020.

Plan A3 – Target Kerala PSC Crash Course (Validity 90 Days)
• **60+** Subject-wise/Grand Tests with Rationale
• **320+** E-Notes in the form of Subject-wise synopsis
• **50+** Hours of Videos in English (Important Topics Pre-loaded video + Chanting videos)
• In association with our Best-Selling Title- Target High Staff Nurse Entrance Exam

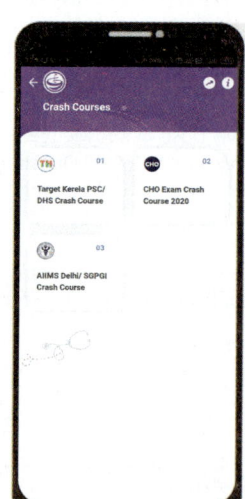

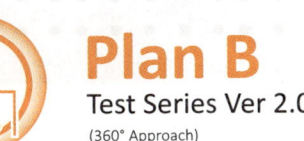

Plan B
Test Series Ver 2.0
(360° Approach)

...t Series Version 2.0 is based on 2 important principles 1) **PRACTICE, PRACTICE & PRACTICE 2) 360° Approach**

...any and all exams from Basics to Advanced Level, keeping in mind the current and probable exam pattern.
...e exam level is upgrading, that's why your preparation also needs to level up!
...e main focus of Test Series Ver 2.0 is to provide you the complete knowledge & preparation in the form of All
...bjects/All Topics' Test, E-Notes, IBQs & VBQs, a variety of New Grand Tests based on Real-Time Exam Pattern of All
...tional & State Level Exams prepared by the experts. To give complete touch to the preparation, we have
...ered All important National & State Level- Most Recent/Previous Year Papers of last 15 years along with Imp
...ics/Exam Discussions Videos

...n:
... provide complete preparation in the form of Tests, E-Notes & through Important Topics Videos
... keep you always prepared and ready for all upcoming exams
...n the principles of Practice makes a person perfect!

...t for:
...hose who do not choose the shortcut way and want to directly go for extensive preparation for any
...taff nurse entrance exam.
...tudents who are well-versed with theoretical concepts of all Subjects but want to upgrade
...nd assess their knowledge to keep themselves abreast with the latest exam pattern and future
...ends.
...tudents who are associated with any online or offline coaching institute, working in hospitals
...r undergraduate, and do not want to compromise with their preparation and success

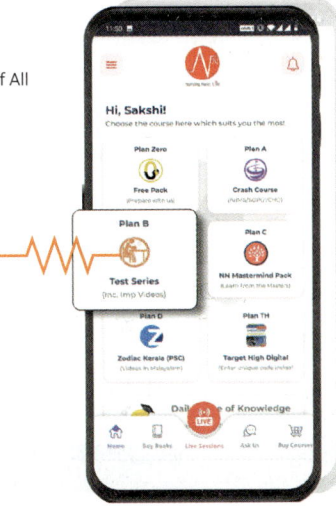

...hat all you will get

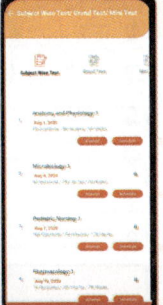

Plan B 2 Test Series (Validity- 6+3 Month) Pre Loaded Content Phase -1
- **90+** Newly Created Subject-wise, Mini Test and Grand Test focusing all important National Exams AIIMS, PGIMER, JIPMER, DSSSB, RRB and ESIC (In 6 Months)
- **6500+** Qs (MCQs, IBQs, VBQs) with Rationale and updated reference from standard textbooks. All the Tests are designed by the Subject Experts and Topper Students (In 6 Months)
- **200+** Hours Recorded Video Lectures of Nursing/Non-Nursing Subjects by some of India's best nursing faculties/subject experts. Lectures are in English/Hindi language focusing on concept-based learning.
- **5** Exam Discussion Videos of 2019 Exam papers (Duration 20 Hours)
- **150+** Hours of Recorded Video on Subject-wise Exam Discussion of previous years papers (2017-18) of all nursing exams delivered by subject experts
- **5** Skill Procedure videos demonstrating Nursing Skills in real-time
- **100+** Previous Year Exam Papers of all Nursing Exams from 2020-10 with Rationale (Attempt/View PDF Mode)
- **1500+** Flash cards on all the important topics of all the subjects for last minute revision (In 6 months)
- **800+** Image-based Questions with Rationale
- **150+** Video-based Qs with Rationale

...se 2 : New subject wise/Mini/Grand Test & Clinical Gems Added as per the pattern of AIIMS NORCET (March - August 21)

...1 Test subject-wise, System wise, Mini Test & Grand Test
...00+ Qs (MCQs, IBQs, VBQs) with Rationale and updated reference from standard textbooks. All the Tests
...e designed by the Subject Experts and Topper Students (In 6 Months)
...0+ Clinical gems of most important topics of different subjects.
...w System wise approach for Medical Surgical Nursing, Pediatric Nursing, Pharmacology, Anatomy and Physiology.
... the content is developed primarily focusing on upcoming AIIMS NORCET 2021 exam by our expert team
... the topics are covered **System-wise** covering following subjects: Medical Surgical Nursing, Pediatric Nursing,
...armacology, Anatomy and Physiology.
...rious Subject-wise tests are also covered individually.
...w Features: Syllabus covered in the various tests will be pre-announced monthly

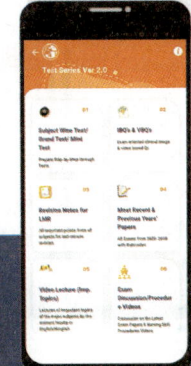

...an BE ESIC Special Mini Test Series (Validity -90 Days)
...omplete access to Plan B for 90 days
... Grand Test and 10 Subject wise tests focusing on ESIC Exam
...0 Previous year ESIC exam papers
... Videos

Plan C / C PLUS

Nursing Next MASTERMIND Pack
(One-in-All, All-in-One)

Nursing Next MASTERMIND Pack is a One-stop destination for complete preparation! Plan C plus is a 'Total Package' that provides 100% preparation for all nursing competitive exams using a futuristic approach and giving nothing but the best. The complete content of this pack is created by the TOP Educators of India, who are the masterminds of their subjects.

It covers All Subjects/All Topics Conceptual Videos, Micro Topic wise MCQs with Rationale, IBQs & VBQs Discussion Videos, Live Doubt Sessions & Rapid Revision Videos before exams. NN Mastermind Pack is a gradual Phase-wise learning journey with the option of Individual and Combined Pack, and a validity period of 12 months!

Plan C plus pack also includes Plan A, Plan B & Plan C (Subject) that ultimately provides you complete preparation for all the nursing competitive exams.

Aim:
• Nothing Beyond this! It provides you the complete preparation from theoretical to practical learning.
• The aim is to provide quality education through conceptual learning and not just to train you
  to crack the exams.
• Helping you at every stage of your preparation through guidance & counseling, study plans, tips & tricks &
  motivational videos.

Best for:
• All the Students who want to have a strong foundation and dreaming of a successful career in nursing.
• Those who are looking for quality guidance from the top faculties of National repute
• Working professionals who want to upgrade their knowledge or still aiming for Staff Nurse Entrance exam, and also
  Nursing Undergraduates who are aiming for Staff Nurse exams.

Plan C Plus - Includes Plan A, B & C (Validity 12 Months)

Special Features
• Nursing Next's **"Mastermind Pack"**, is a **One-Stop solution** for all your exam preparation needs for Staff
  Nurse Entrance Exams & Nursing Undergraduate Exams!
• It is our **One-in-All, All-in-One** pack for the nursing students of the Digital era!
• NN Mastermind Pack is exactly that 'learning tool' for all the nursing aspirants. It is carefully planned, and
  strategically designed, under the expertise of TOP Medical/Nursing Educators, just to make learning more
  authentic and easier for our students.
• Covering All Subjects, All Topics concepts from **Basics to Advanced level** pattern with the help of
  Videos/Question Bank & Handwritten Notes
• The Masterminds (TOP EDUCATORS) of NN Live have focused on ALL the upcoming **Nursing Exams** by giving
  two convenient options under 'Individual Subject Pack', & 'Combined (NN Mastermind Pack)'
• **NN Mastermind** Pack is a "road to success" for those who are preparing for any or all **staff nurse entrance
  exams.**

What all you will get

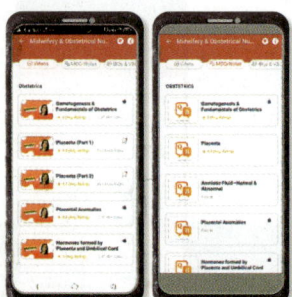

Plan C plus (Inc. Plan A + Plan B + Plan C)
• **1200+** hours of Video Lectures on All Subject/All Topics
• **11,000+** Questions with Rationale covering All Subject/All Topics
• IBQs/VBQs Video Discussions of All Subjects
• **Monthly Live Doubt Sessions**
• Rapid Revision Videos for AIIMS NORCET 2021 (June)
• Handwritten Notes of videos in PDF form will be integrated in the app by Feb/Mar '21
• Focusing on Quality study over quantity study, using the smart-study approach
• All the Content will be Live in Four Phases in 4 Months (Nov-Feb '21)
• Monthly Mega Assessment Tests as per AIMS Norcet 2021 pattern prepared by Mastermind Faculty
• All upcoming exams Important Topics & Exam/Discussions will be covered
• Complete 360 Approach for preparation
• Unlimited Watch Time, FREE Download Video option, National Level Ranks,
   Bookmark the content, Pause & Resume
• Best Guidance & Support at every stage
   + Plan A of NN Live (Complete access to Current & Upcoming Crash Courses)
   + Plan B of NN Live (Complete access to Test Series Version 2.0)
   Refer to Plan A, B, & C for more details, on the content included with Plan C plus

The Masterminds

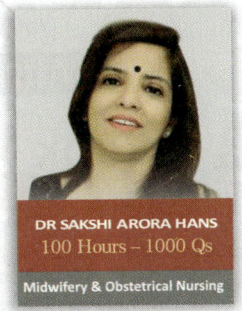

DR SAKSHI ARORA HANS
100 Hours – 1000 Qs
Midwifery & Obstetrical Nursing

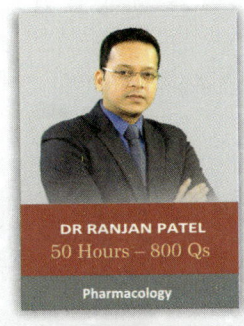

DR ROHAN KHANDELWAL
50 Hours – 600 Qs
MSN-Surgery

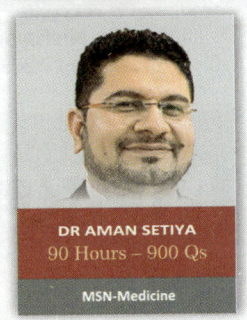

DR RANJAN PATEL
50 Hours – 800 Qs
Pharmacology

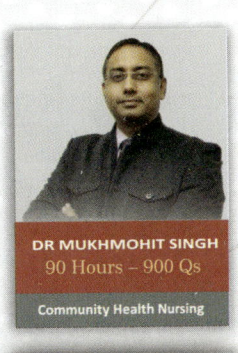

DR MUKHMOHIT SINGH
90 Hours – 900 Qs
Community Health Nursing

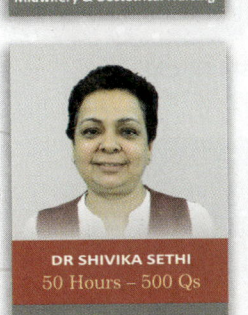

DR SHIVIKA SETHI
50 Hours – 500 Qs
Microbiology

DR ASHISH KUMAR
60 Hours – 600 Qs
Physiology

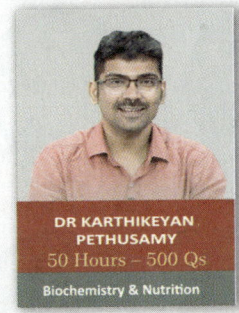

DR AMAN SETIYA
90 Hours – 900 Qs
MSN-Medicine

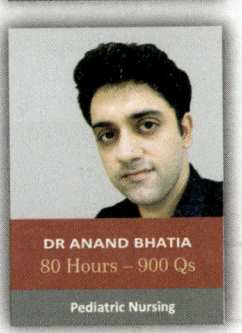

DR ANAND BHATIA
80 Hours – 900 Qs
Pediatric Nursing

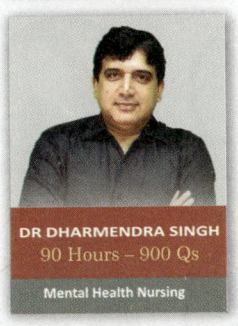
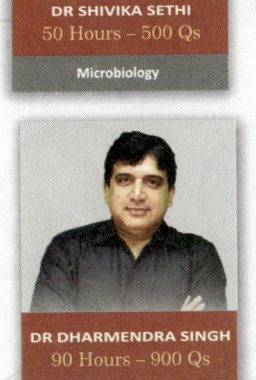

DR DHARMENDRA SINGH
90 Hours – 900 Qs
Mental Health Nursing

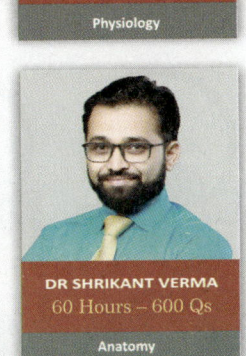
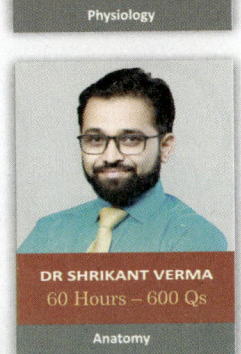

DR SHRIKANT VERMA
60 Hours – 600 Qs
Anatomy

DR KARTHIKEYAN PETHUSAMY
50 Hours – 500 Qs
Biochemistry & Nutrition

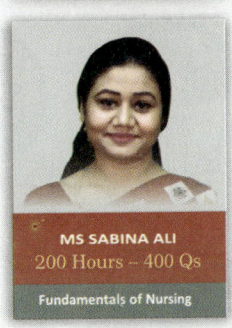

MS SABINA ALI
200 Hours – 400 Qs
Fundamentals of Nursing

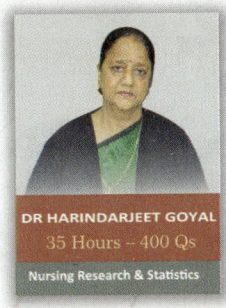

DR HARINDARJEET GOYAL
35 Hours – 400 Qs
Nursing Research & Statistics

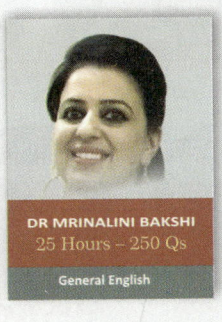

DR MRINALINI BAKSHI
25 Hours – 250 Qs
General English

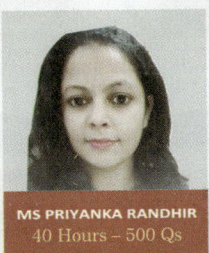
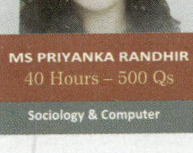

MS PRIYANKA RANDHIR
40 Hours – 500 Qs
Sociology & Computer

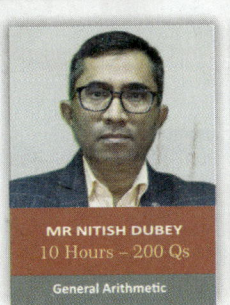

MR NITISH DUBEY
10 Hours – 200 Qs
General Arithmetic

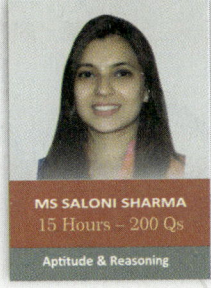

MS SALONI SHARMA
15 Hours – 200 Qs
Aptitude & Reasoning

TOP RANK HOLDERS

With over 300+

Say Hello to the
You car

AIIMS

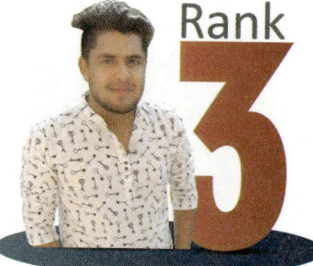

Rank 3
Rahul Dahiya
Roll No. 9016060

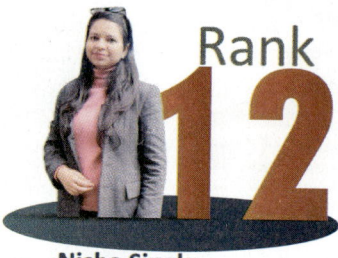

Rank 12
Nisha Singla
Roll No. 9101820

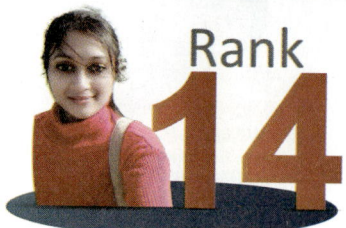

Rank 14
Arushi Mittal
Roll No. 9079646

NORCET 2020

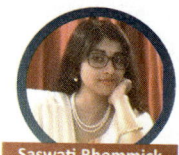
Saswati Bhommick
Rank - 141
Roll No. 9012620

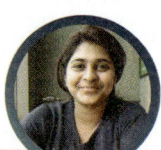
Sohini Mandal
Rank - 145
Roll No. 9042723

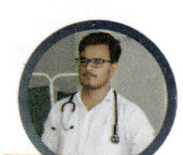
Divyanshu Khandelwal
Rank - 152
Roll No. 9011121

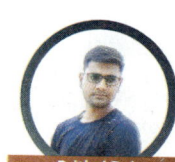
Prithvi Raj
Rank - 171
Roll No. 9030852

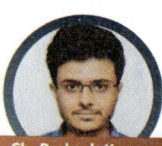
Ch. Prakash Kumar Nanjibhai
Rank - 244
Roll No. 9057267

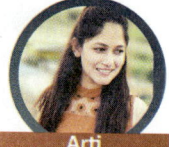
Arti
Rank- 245
Roll No. 9090452

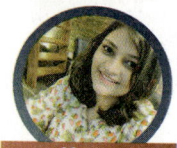
Mamta
Rank- 297
Roll No. 9063879

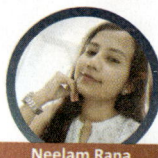
Neelam Rana
Rank- 326
Roll No. 9089800

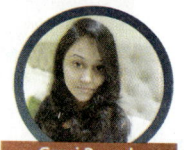
Gargi Baruah
Rank- 336
Roll No. 9019608

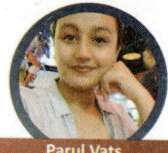
Parul Vats
Rank- 338
Roll No. 9027211

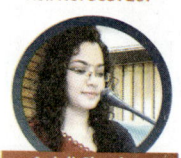
Anjali Chauhan
Rank- 367
Roll No. 9053536

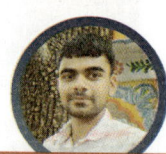
Vishal Gupta
Rank- 384
Roll No. 9023854

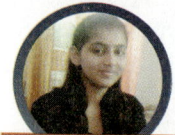
Annu Dahiya
Rank - 390
Roll No. 9005214

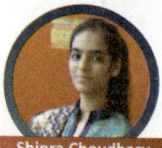
Shipra Choudhary
Rank - 417
Roll No. 9049237

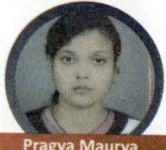
Pragya Maurya
Rank - 466
Roll No. 9033415

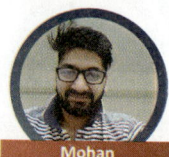
Mohan
Rank - 498
Roll No. 9090721

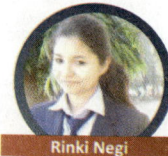
Rinki Negi
Rank - 519
Roll No. 9004223

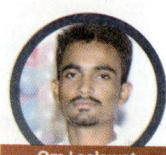
Om Leelawat
Rank - 523
Roll No. 9025575

# of Nursing Next Live

Various National/State Level Exams

NursingNext Squad!
be the next!

NORCET 2020

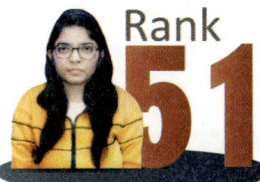
Rank **51**
Komal Dhull
Roll No. 9024458

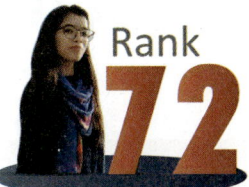
Rank **72**
Shivani Bourai
Roll No. 9092877

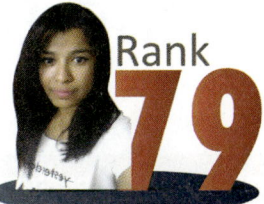
Rank **79**
Nivedita Saini
Roll No. 9004587

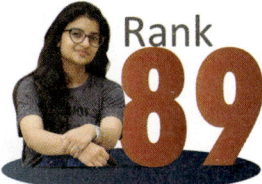
Rank **89**
Rupali Garg
Roll No. 9054544

CHO Selection

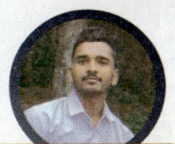
Suresh Kumsr
Rank- 1
Roll No. 12090
MP

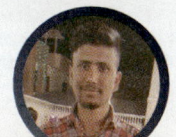
Vikas Kumar Sahu
Rank- 14
Roll No. 10011
MP

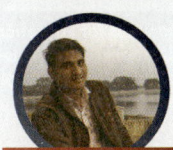
Harish Kumar Lodha
Rank- 18
Roll No. 7930
MP

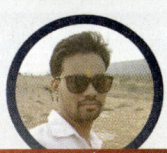
Heeralal Lodha
Rank- 33
Roll No. 10009
MP

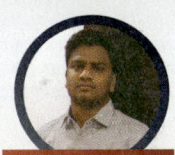
Sandeep Krumar Kumawat
Rank- 44
Roll No. 12585
MP

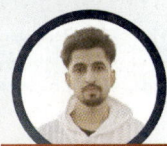
Mahadev Aanjan
Rank- 50
Roll No. 10130
MP

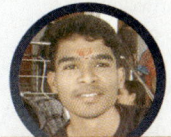
Nilesh
Rank- 81
Roll No. 10572
MP

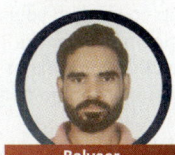
Balveer
Roll No. 619175
RAJASTHAN

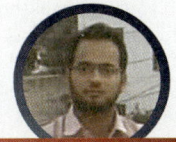
Mahendra Singh Gurjar
Roll No. 626167
RAJASTHAN

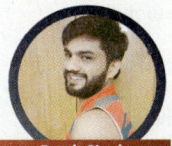
Fateh Singh
Roll No. 108169
RAJASTHAN

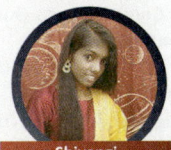
Shivangi
Roll No. 406105
RAJASTHAN

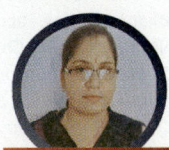
Suneeta Swami
Roll No. 619378
RAJASTHAN

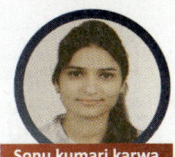
Sonu kumari karwa
Roll No. 600665
RAJASTHAN

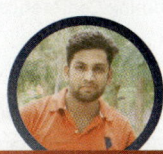
Vikram prakash kumhar
Roll No. - 301468
RAJASTHAN

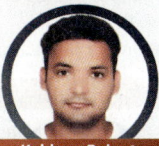
Kuldeep Rajput
Roll No. 407675
RAJASTHAN

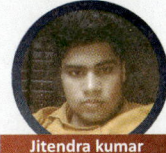
Jitendra kumar
Roll No. 614378
RAJASTHAN

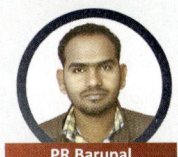
PR Barupal
Roll No. 100261
RAJASTHAN

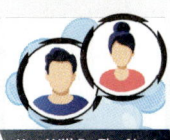
You Will Be The Next...

AN INVITATION TO ALL THE NURSING FACULTY MEMBERS TO COME

JOIN US NOW!

Nursing Next SOCIAL

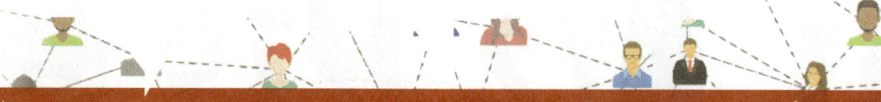

India's first networking platform for the Exclusively Nursing Segment!

GAINING KNOWLEDGE IS THE FIRST STEP TO WISDOM, SHARING IT... IS THE FIRST STEP TO HUMANITY!

Nursing Next Live has come out with one more initiative of bringing all the Nursing Faculties from across the nation Closer & Together on a Single Platform.

Now, distance will not be a barrier. All the Faculties from Kashmir to Kanyakumari will be at one platform. We have come out with a revolutionary idea called "Nursing Next Live Social" to connect...
ALL NURSING FACULTIES FROM ALL STATES & ALL SEGMENTS TOGETHER!

Rewards For You

- Get Acknowledgement & Appreciation Certificates • Get Sponsorships for Educational Programs, Conferences & Webinars!
- Get Free Access to Nursing Next Live Content & CBS Nursing Books • Get Latest Updates related to your subject
- Get a chance to become Reviewer, Contributors in Nursing Next Live, Target High & in CBS Nursing Titles

BE THE MENTOR OR MENTEE
SHOWCASE YOUR ACHIEVEMENTS ➡ SHARE YOUR KNOWLEDGE

Purposes:
- To link all the Nursing Faculties Together and make a strong Nursing Faculty Community as One Nation One Nursing Faculty Community
- To provide a Platform where all the faculties can showcase their accomplishments
- Conducting Various Scientific Activities for knowledge upgradation

Special Features
- Create Your Profile
- Add your accomplishments to level up your portfolio
- Earn Reward Points & Redeem through various options
- Set your Professional GOALS with Timelines
- Be the part of active discussions related to Nursing and provide your valuable inputs
- Attend Complimentary Webinars & Scientific Programs
- Explore various job & career growth opportunities
- Give your reviews & ratings on Books & Colleges
- Regular Updates on upcoming Conferences, CNE & Webinars
- Become a Mentor or Mentee

Scan the QR Code &
Fill the form to Pre-Register

PRE-REGISTER FOR NURSING NEXT SOCIAL
& Get 60 Days Free Subscription of Nursing Next Live App

ARE YOU A NURSING FACULTY ?
BE THE PART OF NURSING NEXT LIVE SOCIAL!

OR Use the below link to fill the for
http://bit.ly/2K4Czq

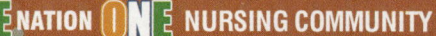
ONE NATION ONE NURSING COMMUNITY

For more details and special offers log on to www.nursingnextlive.com

Make Your Students GenNext

The Smart Digital Library

Future Ready Students
Make your students stand out from the crowd

With the help of Smart Digital Library you can upgrade the knowledge and skills of students and make them ready as per the current and future trends in competitions

Extra Knowledge
Give your students the content beyond their regular course

Inspire your students to learn extra so that they always stay ahead in all competitive exam

Going with the Trend
Go Digital- Be a trend setter

Traditional libraries are now being replaced by Smart Libraries. Act as the pioneer of this change and give your institute and students the best e-resource

Increased Brand Value of your Institution
Create a prominent place among other institutes

Enhance your institute's brand value with the help of Smart Digital Library and let us build the image of your institution together as a quality and technologically advanced education provider

Cost- & Time-Effective
Utilise your money and resources in constructive works

Smart Digital Libraries store much more information in a little physical space with much lower cost. Also, readily available learning e-resources with handy test results eliminate the paper-based system, and manual checking which consumes a lot of time of faculty

What all you will get?

- Complete access to all the Content of all Courses (Crash Courses, Test Series Ver 2.0, Mastermind Pack) with Unlimited Watch Time & the option of re-attempting test.
- All Topics of All Subjects (as per INC syllabus) are covered in form of Video Lectures, MCQs with Rationales, E-Notes, Hand Written Notes (PDF form will be integrated in the app by Feb '21) & Subjective Qs along with IBQs, VBQs, Most Recent & Previous Year Papers, and Live Doubt Sessions per month with Faculties.
- New Content will be added every month. Therefore, the Quantity of your Content will increase gradually throughout your subscription period.
- Regular Online Training Sessions for Best Guidance & Support on "How to Prepare for Nursing Competitive Exams" from the Top experts.
- Get a Dashboard to monitor your Students Progress Chart and Total Usage. *(Forthcoming)*
- Smart Digital Library is available in 2 versions 1) Tablet Version 2) Desktop Application Version.
- Avail Best Discounts & Special Offers on Smart Digital Library. The Institutional Subscription starts with a minimum of 20 subscriptions

For Business Proposal-related enquiries, contact:

Bhupesh Arora (Project Director)
+91-9555590180
bhupesharora@nursingnextlive.in

Jogendra Singh (Sr. Business Developement Manager)
+91-9311866854
jogendra@nursingnextlive.in

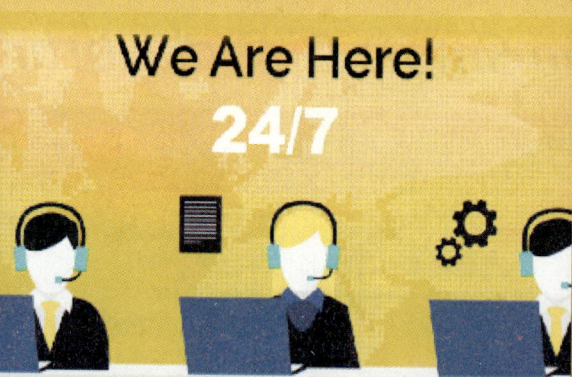

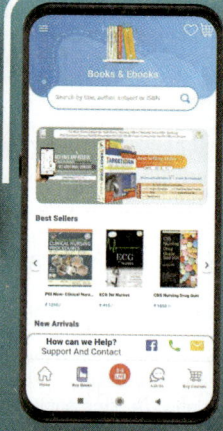
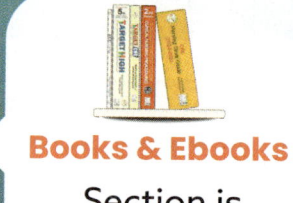
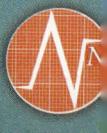

Textbook of

Microbiology

for GNM Nursing Students

(As per new syllabus of INC for GNM)

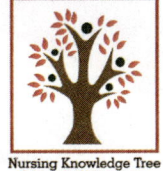

Nursing Knowledge Tree
An Initiative by CBS Nursing Division

Second Edition

Mrinalini Bakshi

Edited by

Indarjit Walia

Anju Dhir

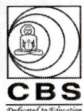

CBS
Dedicated to Education

CBS Publishers & Distributors Pvt Ltd

• New Delhi • Bengaluru • Chennai • Kochi • Kolkata • Mumbai
• Hyderabad • Nagpur • Patna • Pune • Vijayawada

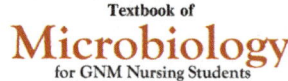

Textbook of
Microbiology
for GNM Nursing Students

ISBN: 978-93-90619-12-2

Second Edition: 2021

First Edition: 2018

Published by **Satish Kumar Jain** and produced by **Varun Jain** for
CBS Publishers & Distributors Pvt Ltd

4819/XI Prahlad Street, 24 Ansari Road, Daryaganj, New Delhi 110 002, India.
Ph: +91-11-23289259, 23266861, 23266867   Website: www.cbspd.com
Fax: 011-23243014
e-mail: delhi@cbspd.com; cbspubs@airtelmail.in.

Corporate Office: 204 FIE, Industrial Area, Patparganj, Delhi 110 092
Ph: +91-11-4934 4934   Fax: 4934 4935
e-mail: feedback@cbspd.com; bhupesharora@cbspd.com

Branches

- **Bengaluru:** Seema House 2975, 17th Cross, K.R. Road, Banasankari 2nd Stage,
  Bengaluru 560 070, Karnataka
  Ph: +91-80-26771678/79   Fax: +91-80-26771680   e-mail: bangalore@cbspd.com

- **Chennai:** 7, Subbaraya Street, Shenoy Nagar, Chennai 600 030, Tamil Nadu
  Ph: +91-44-26680620, 26681266   Fax: +91-44-42032115   e-mail: chennai@cbspd.com

- **Kochi:** 68/1534, 35, 36-Power House Road, Opp. KSEB, Cochin-682018, Kochi, Kerala
  Ph: +91-484-4059061-65   Fax: +91-484-4059065   e-mail: kochi@cbspd.com

- **Kolkata:** 6/B, Ground Floor, Rameswar Shaw Road, Kolkata-700 014, West Bengal
  Ph: +91-33-22891126, 22891127, 22891128   e-mail: kolkata@cbspd.com

- **Mumbai:** 83-C, Dr E Moses Road, Worli, Mumbai-400018, Maharashtra
  Ph: +91-22-24902340/41   Fax: +91-22-24902342   e-mail: mumbai@cbspd.com

Representatives

- **Hyderabad**   +91-9885175004   • **Patna**   +91-9334159340
- **Pune**   +91-9623451994   • **Vijayawada**   +91-9000660880

Printed at: Goyal Offset Works Pvt. Ltd.

Preface

Microbes, the most abundant form of life, are invisible to naked eyes and affect almost every aspect of our lives. Nurses being an integral part of Preventive Medicine and Healthcare, it becomes imperative for them to study microbiology as they are involved with patient care in hospitals and take part in community health teachings to educate communities. Moreover, they need to protect themselves so as to avoid catching any infections while serving humanity. To achieve the goal of self protection against diseases and to look after patient in perfect hygienic way, knowledge of microbiology is a must.

The second edition of this book has been developed as per the latest syllabus of Indian Nursing Council (INC) for General Nursing and Midwifery (GNM) students to help them understand the subject in most concise yet comprehensive manner. The contents have been arranged in a way so that all the important and practical aspects of microbiology from nursing perspective could be well-dealt in simple and easy-to-understand language.

The second edition of this book have been updated as per the recent advancement in the relevant field of nursing till now. Most approaching feature of the book is separate updates on COVID, covering all the details about it. In this edition relevant diagrams, images and tables have been added to illustrate the text in a lucid and vivid manner. The text is supported by boxes, like "Terms to Learn" (contain the meanings of important terms coming across in the continued chapter) and "Also Know" (contain additional important information related to the topic under discussion to read).

Every chapter ends with "Assess Yourself" section that contains multiple choice questions along with their correct answers for helping the students to assess their understanding after studying the chapter. The present edition contains plenty of MCQs which have been extracted from previous year examination papers. Color Plates have been added for common bacterial, viral, fungal disease, etc. to portray real pictures of the diseases. This book has been developed sincerely with an aim of simplifying the subject for the readers and it is hoped that it suffices the needs of the GNM students. Although utmost care has been taken while developing the book, the possibility of some inadvertent errors that may have crept in, could not be denied.

I will be extremely grateful to receive the feedback for improvement as "There is no end to the journey towards perfection". I sincerely hope that you would experience the same pleasure in reading this book as I experienced while developing it.

Mrinalini Bakshi

Acknowledgments

"Feeling gratitude and not expressing it is like wrapping a present and not giving it."

—*William Arthur Ward*

The completion of this book is not the effort of one person. It is the fruit of efforts and beliefs of many who have influenced me and made me capable to accomplish this task.

To begin with, I would like to express my gratitude to the pillars of my life, my mother, **Mrs Nalini Bakshi**, my father, **Mr Brijender Kumar Bakshi** and brother, **Vikram**. You are a family to live for and die for. You people are the constant stream of strength for me and I am glad that I have been nurtured with the selfless love you all have offered. I consider myself God's favorite to be blessed with a family like you.

I am grateful to the Almighty for giving me this opportunity to be mentored and sculpted in the hands of **Dr Ramakant Jagpal**, who has been an inspiration in my struggles and who infused the "never-say-die" attitude in me. This is the beginning of my *Guru Dakshina* to you. I fall short of words to thank **Dr Manish Jagpal** and **Dr Amar Jagpal**, for believing in me and making me explore the various dimensions of my capabilities. You are the reason I never gave up and always strived to explore and learn more.

I am thankful to **Dr Indarjit Walia**, a humble figure, for guiding me through the making of this book and accepting the responsibility of editing this compendium. It was her support and vision that gave this book its present outlook.

I am again thankful to **Dr Anju Dhir** for editing second edition of this book. She has updated this edition thoroughly and helped me to present it in this form.

I am extremely thankful to **Dr Sakshi Arora Hans**, who is the reason why I developed this interest. You have no idea how much instrumental you have been in shaping my career and today if I am able to develop this book, it is because of you. I thank you for inspiring me to learn and develop my skills further.

I cannot thank enough the person who has faced the worst of my outbursts but never failed to believe in me, my friend, **Himanshu**. Thank you for standing by me in the worst of my times and going beyond limits to keep me focused and motivated for accomplishing things.

This book would never have been a reality without the belief and support of two most important people, **Mr Satish Kumar Jain** (Chairman) and **Mr Varun Jain** (Managing Director), M/s CBS Publishers and Distributors Pvt Ltd. I am thankful to them for their immense encouragement and guidance in the publication of this book. One more person who has acted like the backbone to this book is **Mr Bhupesh Arora** (Vice President – Publishing & Marketing, PGMEE & Nursing Division), without him this book wouldn't have been what it is today.

I acknowledge the entire CBS Team for creating an amazing layout for the book and playing an instrumental role in presentation of the content in the best possible manner. I cannot thank Ms Nitasha Arora (Production Head & Content Strategist) enough for her wholehearted support, cooperation and maintaining patience during the making of this book. Mr Shivendu Bhushan Pandey, Mr Ashutosh Pathak and all the production team members, Mr Phool Kumar, Mr Prakash Gaur, Mr Chaman Lal, Mr Bunty Kashyap, Ms Manorama Gupta, Ms Babita Verma, Mr Chander Mani, Mr Manoj Chaudhary, Mr Arun Kumar and Mr Rahul Negi for putting their hardwork and efforts to bring out this handbook on time.

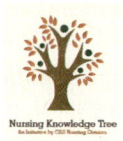

Nursing Knowledge Tree

An Initiative by CBS Nursing Division

"Coming together is a beginning. Keeping together is progress. Working together is success."

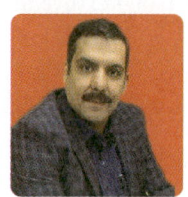

It gives us immense pleasure to share with you that the Nursing Knowledge Tree—An Initiative by CBS Nursing Division, has successfully established itself in the field of nursing as we have been able to stand as a strong contender by sharing approximately 50% of the market share. This growth could not have been possible without your invaluable contribution as our reader, author, reviewer, contributor and recommender, and your outstanding support for the growth of our titles as a whole. You people are the pillars of our series and we are so glad that you all have strengthened our basic foundations.

Nursing Knowledge Tree has been a pioneer and specialist in publishing best quality books for nursing education. Keeping in mind the changing trends in Nursing Education, we at Nursing Knowledge Tree have taken up a mission to bring student friendly and syllabus-based books written by Subject Experts from PAN India.

Our Noteworthy Achievements:
- Our nationally-acclaimed titles
  - *PGIMER NINE Clinical Nursing Procedures*—**Sandhya Ghai**
  - *Target High Staff Nurse Entrance Examination*—**Muthuvenkatachalam S, Ambili M Venugopal**
  - *CBS Nursing Drug Guide*—**Yogesh Gulati/Rakesh Sharma**
  - *Textbook of Nursing Foundations*—**Harindarjeet Goyal**
  - *Essentials of Biochemistry*—**Harbans Lal**
  - *Textbook of Nursing Education*—**Ratna Prakash**
  - *Nursing Research in 21st Century*—**Sukhpal Kaur and Amarjeet Singh**
  - *Essentials of Applied Microbiology*—**DR Arora and Brij Bala Arora**
  - *Textbook of Pediatric Nursing*—**Meharban Singh and Raman Kalia**
- Liaised with the topmost institutes of the country, like **AIIMS, NIMHANS, PGIMER NINE, CMC-Vellore, Manipal University, JIPMER, RAK-Delhi**, etc.
- Published **100+ Quality Nursing Books** and more than **50 New Books** on various subjects for Nursing Undergraduates, Postgraduates and Nursing superspecialty are under process and will be releasing in 2021.
- Increased our social presence by participating more than **200+ National Conferences, CME's, College Exhibitions & Webinars** in previous years.
- We have come out with **Nursing Next Live**, it is an EdTech platform, The Next Level of Nursing Education, where we are bringing learning to people, instead of people going for learning. Through NNL App we are providing various study modules/plans covering All Subjects/All Topics, Video Lectures, Question Bank, E-notes and Variety of Test. Students can choose the plan as per their needs and wants.
- We are exicted to announce that we are coming out with our new initiative—**Nursing Next Live Social**, where nursing faculties can share as well as gain knowledge, with the aim to revolutionize the way the nursing segment connects. It's going to be India's first networking platform for Nursing Segment.

Our Journey towards providing Quality Nursing Education is Incomplete without YOU ! Join Us Now !

We specialize in publishing nursing books of superior quality, going ahead we see us publishing more and more quality content and it will only be possible when intellectuals from across the nation come together. Keeping pace with the advancements, we want to strengthen the nursing sector which was long neglected, and establish a strong foundation when it comes to quality content for the segment.

We are determined to bring about changes in the Nursing Education system and we will do it for sure with your support and contribution. We will be delighted if you join hands with us in the form of Author, Contributor or Reviewer and take the vision of quality education for nursing students ahead.

Let's Join hands together, share your ideas and knowledge with us. Be the part of this Revolution. We are looking forward to your cooperation in future as well. Share your CVs at **bhupesharora@nursingnextlive.in** or scan the given QR code and fill the form or you can talk to me directly at +9811132333.

With Best Wishes
Mr Bhupesh Arora
(Vice President - CBS Nursing Division)

Syllabus for GNM

MICROBIOLOGY

Course Description

This course is designed to help students gain knowledge and understanding of the characteristics and activities of microorganisms, how they react under different conditions and how they cause different disorders and diseases. Knowledge of these principles will enable students to understand and adopt practices associated with preventive and promotive health care.

General Objectives

Upon completion of the course, the students shall be able to:
1. Describe the classifications and characteristics of microorganisms
2. List the common disease producing microorganisms
3. Explain the activities of microorganisms in relation to the environment and the human body
4. Enumerate the basic principles of control and destruction of microorganisms
5. Apply the principles of microbiology in nursing practice.

Total Hours – 30

Unit No.	Learning objectives	Content	Hrs.	Teaching learning activities	Assessment methods
I.	Describe evolution of microbiology and its relevance in nursing	**Introduction** • History of bacteriology and microbiology • Scope of microbiology in nursing	3	Lecture cum discussions	• Objective type • Short answers
II.	• Classify the different types of microorganism • Describe the normal flora and the common diseases caused by pathogens • Explain the methods to study microbes	**Microorganisms** • Classification, characteristics, (structure, size, method and rate of reproduction) • Normal flora of the body • Pathogenesis and common diseases • Methods for study of microbes, culture and isolation of microbes	8	• Lecture cum discussions • Explain using slides, films, videos, exhibits, models • Staining and fixation of slides	• Short answer • Objective type • Essay type

Contd...

Unit No.	Learning objectives	Content	Hrs.	Teaching learning activities	Assessment methods
III.	• Describe the sources of infection and growth of microbes • Explain the transmission of infection and the principles in collecting specimens	**Infection and its Transmission** • Sources and types of infection, nosocomial infection • Factors affecting growth of microbes • Cycle of transmission of infection portals of entry, exit, modes of transfer • Reaction of body to infection, mechanism of resistance • Collection of specimens	4	• Lecture demonstrations • Specimens • Explain using charts	• Short answer • Objective type • Essay type
IV.	Describe various types of immunity, hypersensitivity autoimmunity and immunizing agents	**Immunity** • Types of immunity—innate and acquired • Immunization schedule. Immunoprophylaxis (vaccines, sera etc.) • Hypersensitivity and autoimmunity • Principles and uses of serological tests	5	• Lecture cum discussions • Demonstration on exhibits	• Short answer • Objective type • Essay type

V.	Describe the various methods of control and destruction of microbes	**Control and Destruction of Microbes**
		• Principles and methods of microbial control
		  ▪ Sterilization
		  ▪ Disinfection
		  ▪ Chemotherapy and antibiotics
		  ▪ Pasteurization
		• Medical and surgical asepsis
		• Biosafety and waste management
			5	• Lecture, demonstration on videos
				• Visit to the CSSD
					• Short answer
					• Objective type
					• Essay type

VI.	• Demonstrate skill in handling and care of microscopes • Identify common microbes under the microscope	**Practical Microbiology** • Microscope—Parts, uses, handling and care of microscope • Observation of staining procedure, preparation and examination of slides and smears • Identification of common microbes under the microscope for morphology of different microbes	5	• Lecture, demonstrations • Specimens • Slides	

Contents

COVID-19 UPDATES

WHAT IS COVID-19?

Coronavirus disease (COVID-19) is an infectious disease caused by a newly discovered coronavirus. Most people who fall sick with COVID-19 experience mild to moderate symptoms and recover without special treatment.

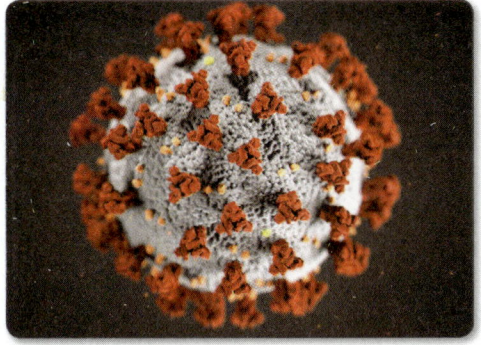

HOW IT SPREADS?

- The virus that causes COVID-19 is mainly transmitted through droplets generated when an infected person coughs, sneezes, or exhales. These droplets are too heavy to hang in the air, and quickly fall on floors or surfaces.
- You can be infected by breathing in the virus if you are within reach of someone who has COVID-19, or by touching a contaminated surface and then your eyes, nose or mouth.

SYMPTOMS

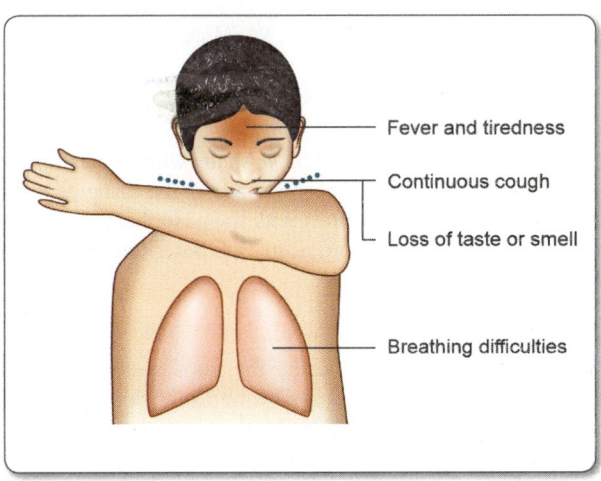

- **Most common symptoms**
  - Fever
  - Dry cough
  - Tiredness
- **Less common symptoms**
  - Aches and pains
  - Sore throat
  - Diarrhea
  - Conjunctivitis
  - Headache
  - Loss of taste or smell
  - A rash on skin, or discoloration of fingers or toes

DIAGNOSIS

At present, polymerase chain reaction (PCR), rapid antigen test and antibody testing are the dominant ways that global healthcare systems are testing citizens for COVID-19.

Sample Collection

Instructions for collecting an Nasopharyngeal (NP) specimen:

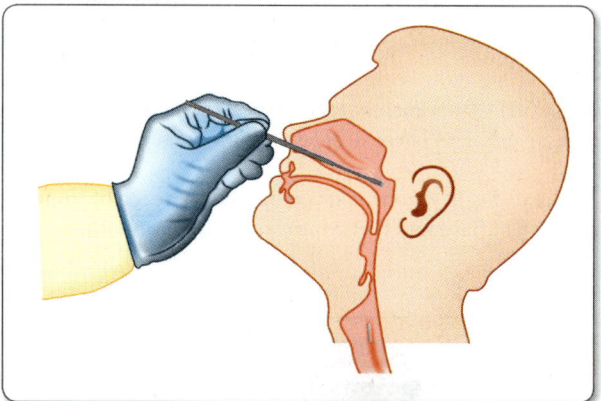

- Tilt patient's head back 70 degrees.
- Gently and slowly insert a minitip swab with a flexible shaft (wire or plastic) through the nostril parallel to the palate (not upwards) until resistance is encountered or the distance is equivalent to that from the ear to the nostril of the patient, indicating contact with the nasopharynx.
- Swab should reach depth equal to distance from nostrils to outer opening of the ear.
- Gently rub and roll the swab.
- Leave swab in place for several seconds to absorb secretions.
- Slowly remove swab while rotating it.
- Specimens can be collected from both sides using the same swab, but it is not necessary to collect specimens from both sides if the minitip is saturated with fluid from the first collection.
- If a deviated septum or blockage creates difficulty in obtaining the specimen from one nostril, use the same swab to obtain the specimen from the other nostril.

Specimen Storage

After collection, store specimens at 2–8°C for up to 72 hours. If a delay in testing or shipping is expected, store specimens at –70°C or below.

For transporting sample: Label each specimen container with the patient's ID number (e.g., medical record number), unique CDC or state-generated nCov specimen ID (e.g., laboratory requisition number), specimen type (e.g., serum) and the date the specimen was collected.

- PCR tests are used to directly detect the presence of an antigen, rather than the presence of the body's immune response, or antibodies.
- **Rapid antigen test:** Rapid antigen tests (sometimes known as a rapid diagnostic test – RDT) detect viral proteins (known as antigens). Samples are collected from the nose and/or throat with a swab as given before.

PREVENTION

- Clean your hands often. Use soap and water, or an alcohol-based hand rub.
- Maintain a safe distance from anyone who is coughing or sneezing.
- Wear a mask when physical distancing is not possible.
- Don't touch your eyes, nose or mouth.
- Cover your nose and mouth with your bent elbow or a tissue when you cough or sneeze.
- Stay home if you feel unwell.
- If you have a fever, cough and difficulty breathing, seek medical attention.

Vaccine

There are three COVID-19 vaccines for which certain national regulatory authorities have authorized the use. None has yet received WHO authorization.

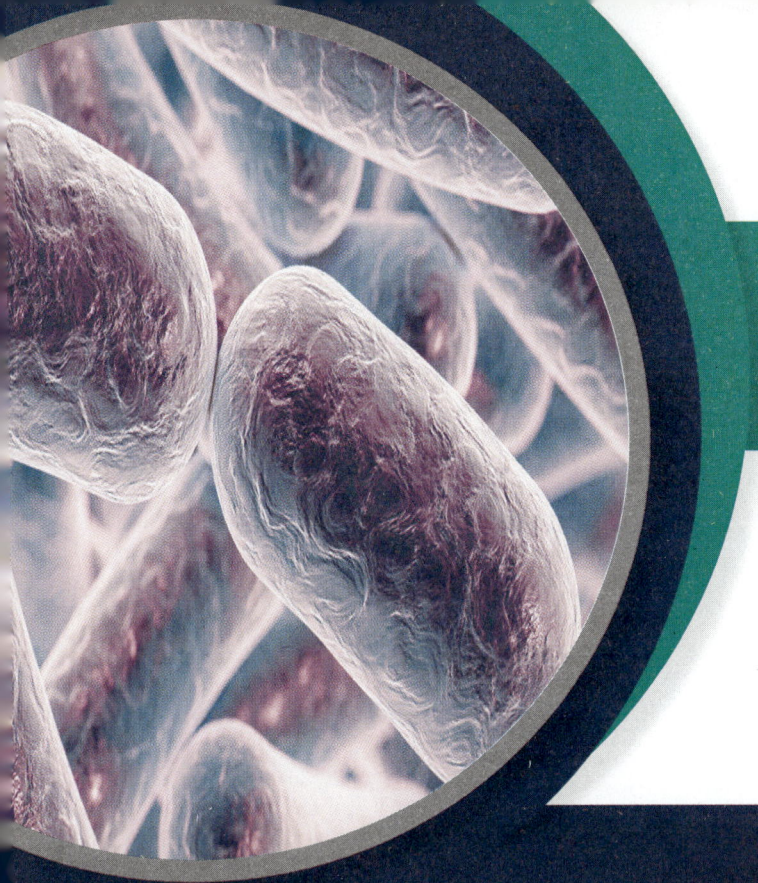

Section I

INTRODUCTION

Microbiology: Historical Introduction and Scope

INTRODUCTION

Microbiology is derived from Greek words; *mikros = small, bios = life, logos = study of*. Thus, microbiology stands for study of those living organisms that are not visible to the naked eye and can be seen only under microscope.

Terms to Learn

- **Bacteriology:** Study of disease causing bacteria
- **Virology:** Study of infectious viruses
- **Mycology:** Study of disease causing fungi
- **Parasitology:** Study of parasites
- **Protozoology:** Study of disease causing protozoans
- **Helminthology:** Study of helminths
- **Nematology:** Study of nematodes

MICROORGANISMS

Microorganisms are not visible to the naked eye and viewed only under microscope. They may be unicellular (having a single cell) or multicellular (having more than one cell).

HISTORICAL PERSPECTIVE

Varo and Columella were the first to give the concept of '*animal minuta*', which stated that diseases are caused by invisible beings after they are inhaled or ingested.

Antonie van Leeuwenhoek (1632–1723)

He is considered to be the 'Father of Microbiology'. He was the first person to see and describe microbes. He gave the term '*animalcules*' for the minute organisms he observed in various samples like rain water and tartar of teeth, under the microscope he developed himself.

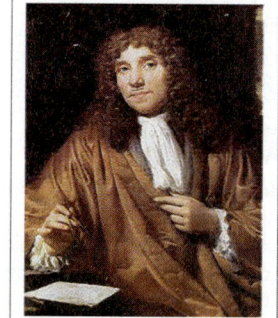

Louis Pasteur (1822–1895)

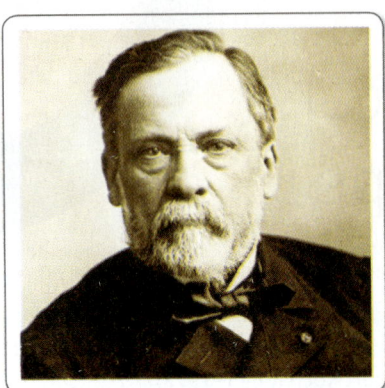

He is considered to be the 'Father of Modern Microbiology'. His important contributions are listed below.

Louis Pasteur – Notable Contributions	
1857	Lactic acid fermentation is due to a microorganism
1860	Yeasts are involved in alcoholic fermentation
1861	Disproved the theory of spontaneous generation
1861	Introduction of the terms aerobic and anaerobic for yeasts. Production of more alcohol in the absence of oxygen during sugar fermentation—**The Pasteur Effect**
1862	Proposed germ theory of disease
1867	Pasteur devised the process of destroying bacteria known as **pasteurization**
1881	Development of anthrax vaccine. Resolved Pebrine problem of silkworms
1885	Development of a special vaccine for rabies (**The Pasteur treatment**)

Terms to Learn

- **Heat-labile bacteria**: Bacteria that can be killed by exposing them to heat
- **Heat-resistant bacteria**: Bacteria that cannot be killed by continuous boiling of the broth
- **Fermentation**: Process that breaks down sugars into alcohol and organic acids

Robert Koch (1843–1912)

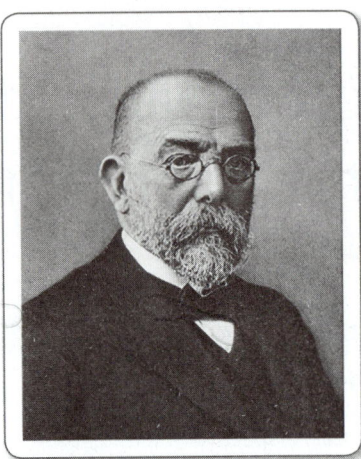

He is regarded as 'Father of Medical Microbiology and Bacteriology'.

Robert Koch – Notable Contributions	
1876	Koch demonstrated that anthrax is caused by *Bacillus anthracis*
1877	Methods for staining bacteria, photographing and preparing permanent visual records on slides
1881	Koch developed solid culture media and the methods for studying bacteria in pure cultures
1882	Isolated the bacterium—*Mycobacterium tuberculosis*—that causes tuberculosis
1882	Use of agar as a support medium for solid culture in Koch's lab by Hesse
1883	Isolation of *Vibrio cholerae*, the cause of cholera
1883	Verification of the germ theory of disease by relating a specific organism to the specific disease
1884	Koch put forth his postulates—known as Koch's postulates

Koch's Postulates

Robert Koch gave the following 4 postulates:

1. The microorganism or other pathogen must be **present in all cases of the disease**.

2. The pathogen can be isolated from the diseased host and **grown in pure culture**.
3. The pathogen from the pure culture must **cause the disease when inoculated into a healthy, susceptible laboratory animal**.
4. The pathogen must be **reisolated** from the new host and **shown to be the same** as the originally inoculated pathogen.

Also Know

Exceptions to Koch's postulates

Treponema pallidum, *Mycobacterium leprae*, many viruses and Rickettsiae are unable to grow on artificial media.

Edward Jenner (1749–1823)

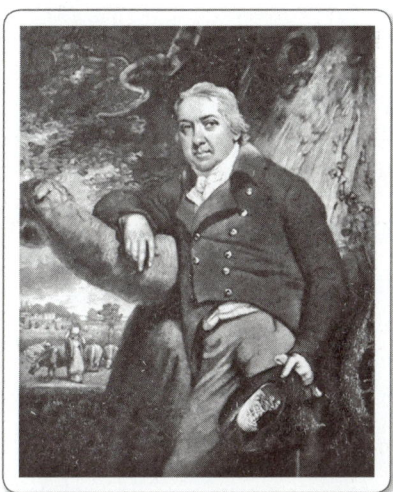

Jenner is known for his discovery that a less pathogenic agent could confer protection against the more pathogenic one, which led to the starting of the era of vaccines and vaccination (discussed in detail in Chapter 13). His greatest gift to the mankind is the cowpox vaccine against smallpox.

Joseph Lister (1827–1912)

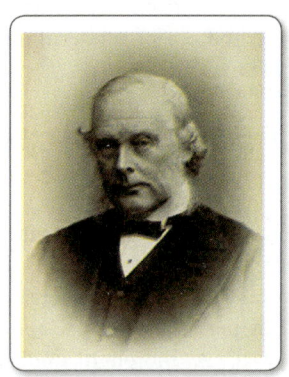

He is known as 'Father of Antiseptic Surgery'. He developed the system of antiseptic surgery in 1867 by being the first person to have used carbolic acid on the wounds during surgery which successfully prevented sepsis. In 1878, he demonstrated the specific cause of milk souring by studying the lactic acid fermentation of milk. He developed method for isolating a pure culture of *Bacterium lactis*.

Alexander Fleming (1881–1955)

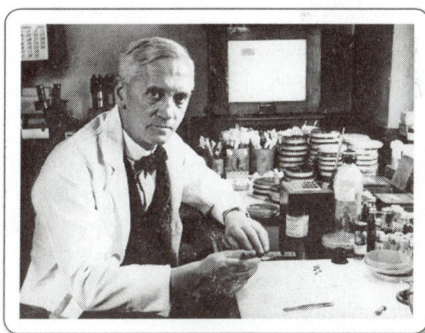

Alexander Fleming, in 1922 discovered that **lysozyme**, an enzyme found in tears, saliva and sweat, could kill bacteria; the first body secretion shown to have chemotherapeutic properties.

He in 1928, made the accidental discovery of first antibiotic, penicillin, from the fungus *Penicillium notatum*. Thus, the era of modern antibiotics was started after Fleming's discovery.

SCOPE OF MICROBIOLOGY IN NURSING

Nurses are an integral part of Preventive Medicine and Healthcare. Understanding of microbiology is very important for nursing professionals as they are involved in personal, hospital and community hygiene as well. A thorough understanding of microbiology is necessary in:

- Understanding the underlying principles of disinfection and sterilization
- Collecting and appropriate handling of specimens
- Identifying pathogenic and non-pathogenic microorganisms
- Interpreting the results in the reports correctly
- Understanding the importance of immunization
- Understanding the susceptibility and resistance of microorganisms to various drugs
- Maintaining hygiene consistent with hospital policies
- Proper monitoring of hospital waste
- Promoting development and improvement of nursing techniques to maintain aseptic environment in the hospital settings.

 Assess Yourself

LONG ANSWER QUESTIONS

1. Write about the Koch's postulates.
2. What is the scope of microbiology for nurses?

SHORT NOTES

1. Louis Pasteur
2. Leeuwenhoek

MULTIPLE CHOICE QUESTIONS

1. Identify correct statement regarding Robert Koch.
   a. He is known as father of bacteriology
   b. The causative organism of cholera, *Vibrio cholera* was identified by him
   c. He discovered hypersensitivity phenomenon
   d. All the above

2. Father of antiseptic surgery is:
   a. Louis Pasteur
   c. Antonie Van Leeuwenhoek
   b. Robert Koch
   d. Joseph Lister

3. Which among the following is a contribution by Louis Pasteur in the field of microbiology?
   a. Techniques of Pasteurization
   c. Rabies, cholera and anthrax vaccine
   b. Process of fermentation
   d. All the above

4. Father of Modern Microbiology is:
   a. Robert Koch
   c. Louis Pasteur
   b. Edward Jenner
   d. Joseph Lister

Contd...

Assess Yourself

5. Who is known as Father of Bacteriology?
   - a. Robert Koch
   - b. Joseph Lister
   - c. Paul Ehrlich
   - d. Antony Van Leeuwenhoek

6. Penicillin was discovered by:
   - a. Robert Koch
   - b. Alexander Fleming
   - c. Joseph Lister
   - d. Antonie van Leeuwenhoek

7. Who discovered antibiotic penicillin?
   - a. Alexander Fleming
   - b. Edward Jenner
   - c. Waksman
   - d. None of these

8. Streptomycin antibiotic was discovered by?
   - a. Alexander flaming
   - b. Waksman
   - c. Frankel
   - d. Neisser

ANSWERS TO MCQS

| 1. d | 2. d | 3. d | 4. c | 5. a | 6. b | 7. a | 8. b |

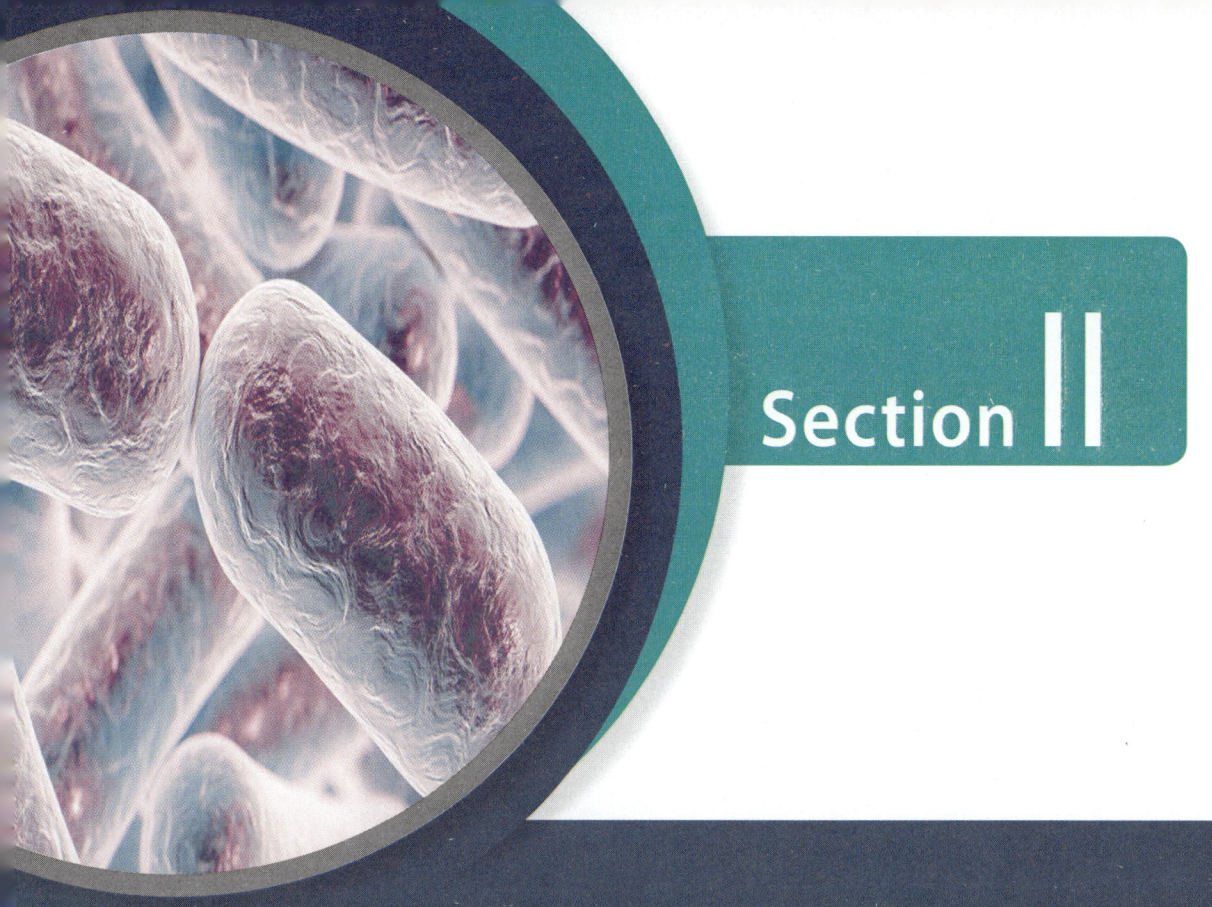

Section II

MICROORGANISMS

Section Summary

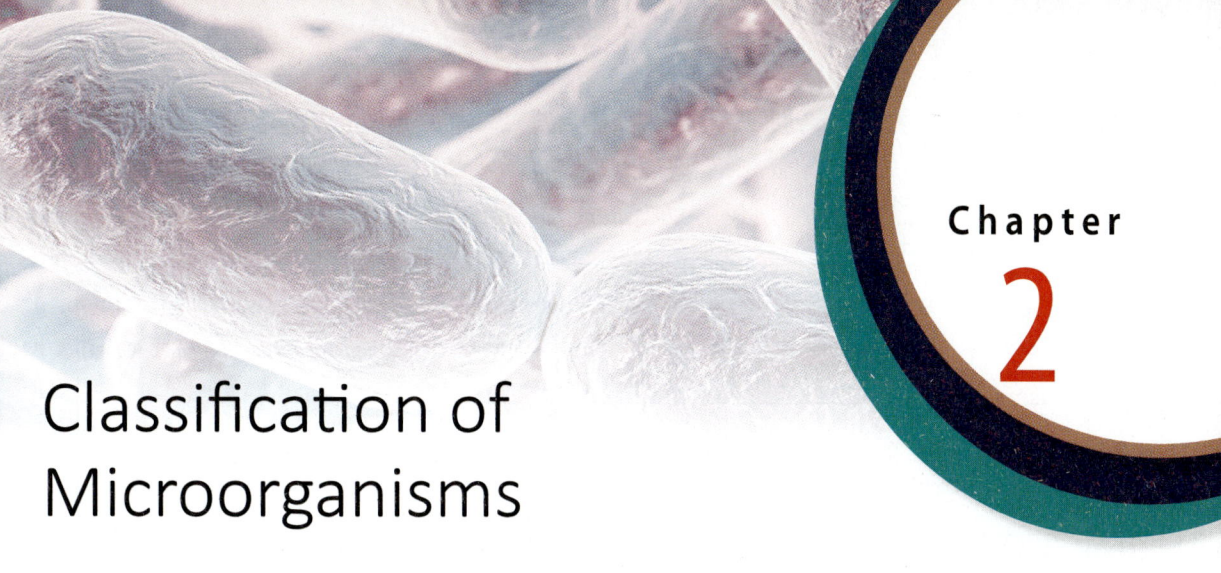

Classification of Microorganisms

INTRODUCTION

Every year, thousands of microorganisms are being discovered and are being added to the already existing list of more than 5 million. Biological classification (taxonomy) is a systematic way of classifying the microorganisms in groups, which share the similar characteristic features.

CLASSIFICATION OF MICROORGANISMS

Microorganisms are classified as follows **(Figure 2.1)**.

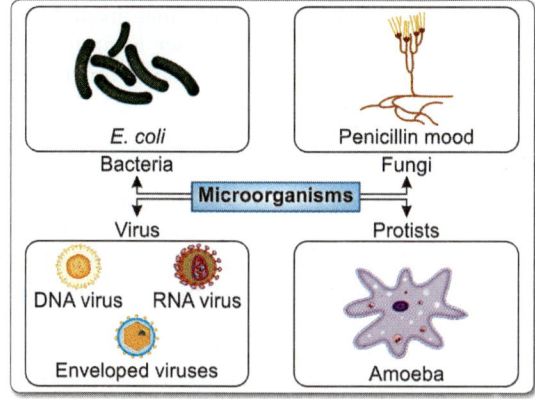

Figure 2.1: Classification of microorganisms

Bacteria

These are single-celled microscopic organisms and measure 0.2–1.5 µm in diameter and 3–5 µm in length. They are classified as **(Figure 2.2)**:

- **Cocci: Spherical bacteria**
  - **Coccus:** Single spherical cells
  - **Diplococcus:** Two spherical cells
  - **Tetrad:** A square of four cells
  - **Sarcina:** A cube of eight cells
  - **Strepotococcus:** Long chain of spherical cells
  - **Staphylococcus:** Grape-like clusters of spherical cells
- **Bacilli: Rod-shaped bacteria**
  - **Bacillus:** Single rod shaped cells
  - **Coccobacillus:** Rod shaped but short and wide enough to look spherical
  - **Palisades:** Loose arrangements along the long edge of the rod
  - **Streptobacillus:** Chains of rod-shaped bacteria
- **Spirilla: Curved or spiral-shaped bacteria**
  - **Vibrios:** Curved rods
  - **Spirillum:** Helical-shaped but rigid
  - **Spirochaete:** Helical-shaped but flexible.

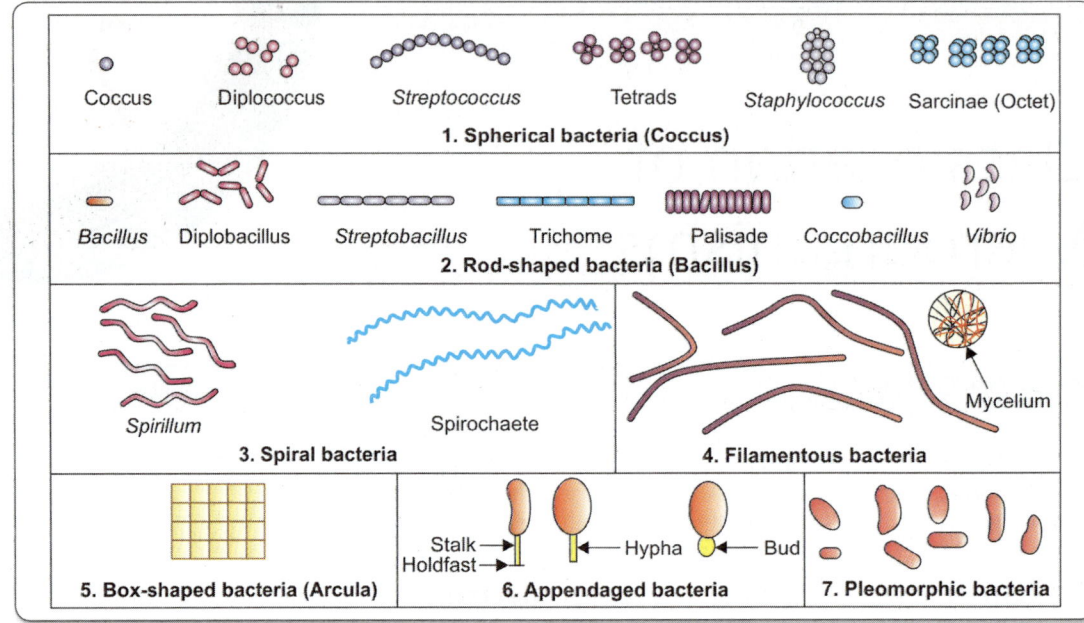

Figure 2.2: Different shapes and arrangements of bacteria

Virus

Viruses are submicroscopic infectious agent that replicate only inside the living cells of an organism. These are visible only under electron microscope. They vary in size from 20 nm to 300 nm. They have either deoxyribonucleic acid (DNA) or ribonucleic acid (RNA) enclosed in a protein coat, called as capsid. They behave as non-living outside the body of host and as living when a suitable host cell is available. The viruses are further classified as given in **Figure 2.3**.

> **Terms to Learn**
>
> • **Virion:** The entire infectious unit of a virus.
> • **Prion:** Infectious particles that are made of only pro-
>   teins and cause diseases of central nervous system.

Protozoa

These are microscopic unicellular microorganisms and are lowest form of animal life. They are larger than bacteria. The pathogenic protozoa are Amoeba, Plasmodium or malarial parasite and Paramecium, etc.

Fungi

Fungi includes unicellular organisms like yeasts and molds and multicellular organisms like mushrooms. They contain chitin in their cell walls that differentiates them from plants and bacteria. They are main decomposers (organisms that break down dead or decaying organisms) in our environment. Examples of common pathogenic fungi are *Candida albicans* and dermatophytes.

Rickettsia

Rickettsia are gram negative, non-spore forming and pleomorphic microorganisms. They may be shaped as minute rods or spheres. They are obligate parasites, i.e. they require a host to sexually reproduce and increase in number. They are generally transmitted to humans by insects and ticks. Typhus and rocky mountain spotted fever are examples of common rickettsial infections.

Enveloped virus			Nonenveloped viruses	
Double-stranded DNA			**Double-stranded DNA**	
Herpesviridae Hepadnaviridae Poxviridae			Adenoviridac Polyomaviridae Papillomaviridae	
			Single-stranded DNA	
			Parvoviridae Circinoviridae	
Single-stranded RNA			**Double-stranded RNA**	
Coronaviridae Paramyxoviridae Bunyaviridae Arenaviridae			Reoviridae	
Orthomyxoviridae Retroviridae Rhabdoviridae			**Single-stranded RNA**	
Togaviridae Flaviviridae Filoviridae			Picornaviridae Caliciviridae	

Figure 2.3: Classification of viruses

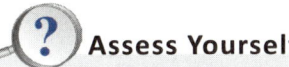

Assess Yourself

LONG ANSWER QUESTION
1. How will you classify microorganisms?

SHORT NOTES
1. Fungi
2. Viruses
3. Protozoa

MULTIPLE CHOICE QUESTIONS
1. Correct regarding cocci are:
   a. Cocci are spherical shaped bacteria
   b. Cocci present in chai n is known as streptococci
   c. Cocci present in the shape of grapes is known as staphylococci
   d. All of the above

Contd...

Assess Yourself

2. Coma-shaped bacteria are known as:
   a. Staphylococci
   b. Streptococci
   c. *Vibrio*
   d. Bacillus

3. The infectious unit of a virus is called:
   a. Prion
   b. Virion
   c. Proton
   d. None of the above

4. Oral and vaginal thrush is caused by:
   a. Trypanosoma
   b. Candida albicans
   c. *Staphylococcus*
   d. All of the above

5. Malarial parasite is a:
   a. Virus
   b. Bacteria
   c. Fungi
   d. Protozoa

6. *Staphylococcus* has:
   a. Single spherical cell
   b. Cube of eight cells
   c. Long chain of spherical cells
   d. Grape-like clusters of spherical cells

ANSWERS TO MCQs

1. d **2.** c **3.** b **4.** b **5.** d **6.** d

Morphology of Bacteria

INTRODUCTION

Bacteria are prokaryotic, single-celled, microscopic organisms. Bacteria are generally much smaller than eukaryotic cells and very complex despite their small size. Structurally, a typical bacterium usually consists of:

- A cytoplasmic membrane surrounded by a peptidoglycan cell wall and maybe an outer membrane
- A fluid cytoplasm containing a nuclear region (nucleoid) and numerous ribosomes
- External structures such as a glycocalyx, flagella, and pili.

Summary of functions of various bacterial cell structures is given in **Table 3.1**.

TABLE 3.1: Summary of Functions of Bacterial Cell Structures

Structure	Function(s)
Flagella	**Swimming movement**
Pili	**Attachment**
Sex pilus	Stabilizes mating bacteria during DNA transfer by conjugation
Common pili or fimbriae	Attachment to surfaces; protection against engulfment
Capsules	Attachment to surfaces; protection against phagocytic engulfment, occasionally killing or digestion; reserve of nutrients or protection against desiccation
Cell wall	**Protection and transfer of nutrients**
Gram-positive bacteria	Prevents osmotic lysis of cell protoplast and confers rigidity and shape on cells
Gram-negative bacteria	Peptidoglycan prevents osmotic lysis and confers rigidity and shape; outer membrane is permeability barrier; associated lipopolysaccharides and proteins have various functions

Contd...

Structure	Function(s)
Plasma membrane	Permeability barrier; transport of solutes; energy generation; location of numerous enzyme systems
Contains cell organelles	
Ribosomes	Sites of translation (protein synthesis)
Inclusions	Often reserves of nutrients; additional specialized functions
Chromosome	Genetic material of cell
Plasmid	Extrachromosomal genetic material

ANATOMY OF A BACTERIAL CELL (FIGURE 3.1)

Flagella

Flagella are filamentous protein structures attached to the cell surface that provide the swimming movement to the bacteria. The diameter of flagellum is about 20 nanometers. The flagellar filament is rotated by a motor apparatus in the plasma membrane allowing the cell to swim in fluid environments. The flagellar apparatus consists of several distinct proteins: A system of rings embedded in the cell envelope (the basal body), a hook-like structure near the cell surface, and the flagellar filament.

The number of flagella and their position on the bacterial cell depends on the species of particular bacteria. They may be **(Figure 3.2)**:

- **Monotrichous:** Bacteria having single polar flagellum
- **Amphitrichous:** When flagella is either single or in clusters at both cell poles

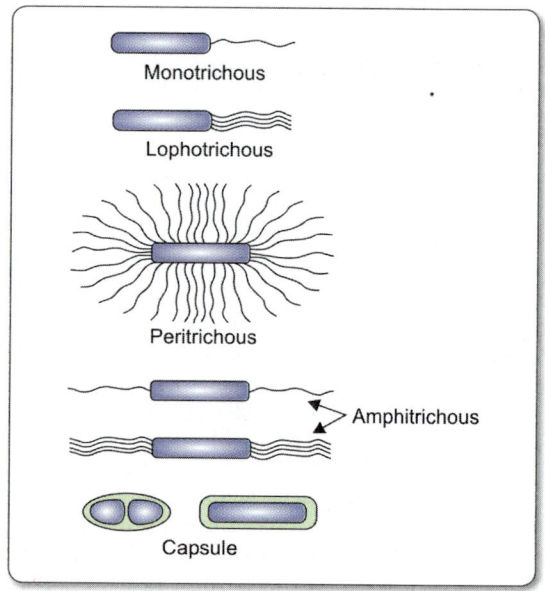

Figure 3.2: Arrangement of bacterial flagella

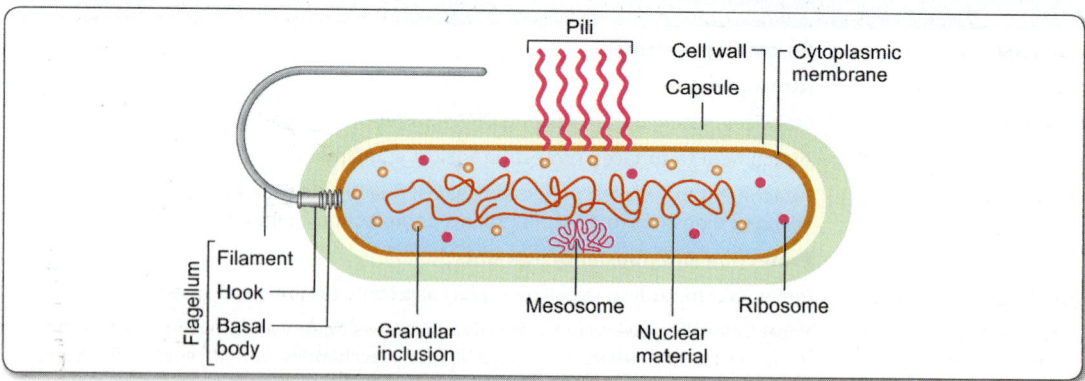

Figure 3.1: Structure of a bacterial cell

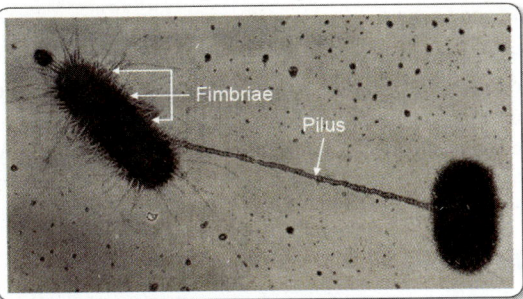

Figure 3.3: Fimbriae and pili of bacteria

TABLE 3.2: Functions of Pili

Bacterial species where observed	Function
Escherichia coli (F or sex pilus)	Stabilizes bacteria during transfer of DNA during conjugation
Escherichia coli (common pili or fimbriae)	Surface adherence to epithelial cells of the gastrointestinal tract
Neisseria gonorrhoeae	Surface adherence to epithelial cells of the urogenital tract
Streptococcus pyogenes (fimbriae plus the M-protein)	Adherence, resistance to phagocytosis; antigenic variability
Pseudomonas aeruginosa	Surface adherence

- **Peritrichous:** When flagella are lateral and surround whole bacteria
- **Lophotrichous:** The flagella are present in the form of a cluster at one pole
- **Atrichous:** When there is no flagellum on the cell.

Fimbriae

Definition: Fimbriae are bristle-like short fibers occur on the surface of some bacteria. Fimbriae enable the bacterial cell to stick to the surface of host cells. They also help in the formation of pellicles or biofilms **(Figure 3.3)**. **(Pellicle:** Thin sheet of cells on the surface of a liquid).

Characteristics

- Fimbriae are bristle-like short fibers.
- Fimbriae are present on both Gram-positive and Gram-negative bacteria.
- Examples of bacteria having fimbriae: *Salmonella typhimurium, Shigella dysenteriae.*
- Fimbriae are made up of **fimbrillin** protein.
- Fimbriae are comparatively shorter in length than pili and flagella.
- Approximate length of fimbriae is 0.03 to 0.14 μm.
- Fimbriae are evenly distributed on the entire surface of the cell.

Pili

Pili definition: Pili are long hair like tubular micro-fibers like structures present on the surface of some Gram-negative bacteria. They are comparatively shorter than flagella and longer than fimbriae. There are many classes of pili based on their structure and function **Table 3.2**.

Characteristics

- Pili are long hair like tubular microfibers like structures.
- Pili are present only on some Gram-negative bacteria.
- Examples of bacteria having pili: *Escherichia coli, Neisseria gonorrhoeae, Pseudomonas.*
- Pili are made up of **pilin** protein.
- Pili are comparatively longer than fimbriae and shorter than flagella.
- Approximate length of pili is 0.5–2 μm.
- Pili are randomly distributed on surface of the cell.
- Number of pili per cell is very less. It usually occurs in the number of 1–10 per cells.
- The formation of pili is controlled by the gene present in plasmids.
- Pili are more rigid than fimbriae.

Capsules

Some bacterial cells are surrounded by a viscous substance forming a covering layer or envelope around the cell wall that is called a capsule. Most bacterial capsules are composed of polysaccharide.

They inhibit the engulfment of pathogenic bacteria by white blood cells (WBCs) and thus contribute to invasive or infective ability known as virulence. They may promote attachment of bacteria to smooth surfaces. Capsule protects the bacteria against ingestion by phagocytes of the host.

Cell Wall

The cell wall is an essential structure that protects the bacteria from mechanical damage and from osmotic rupture or lysis.

- In the Gram-positive bacteria, the cell wall consists of several layers of peptidoglycan. Running perpendicular to the peptidoglycan sheets is a group of molecules called teichoic acids, which are unique to the Gram-positive cell wall.
- The walls of Gram-negative bacteria are more complex as compared to Gram-positive bacteria. There is an outer membrane that surrounds the thin underlying layer of peptidoglycan, rich in lipids. The outer membrane of Gram-negative bacteria invariably contains a unique component, lipopolysaccharide, which is toxic in nature.

Cytoplasmic Membrane

Bacterial membranes are composed of 40% phospholipid and 60% proteins. The phospholipids are amphoteric molecules with a polar hydrophilic glycerol "head" attached via an ester bond to two nonpolar hydrophobic fatty acid tails, which naturally form a bilayer in aqueous environments. Dispersed within the bilayer are various structural and enzymatic proteins, which carry out most membrane functions. Its main function is as a selective permeability barrier that regulates the passage of substances into and out of the cell.

Cytoplasm

It contains ribosomes, mesosomes, vacuoles and inclusions.

Ribosomes

They are the primary sites of protein synthesis and are composed of ribonucleic acid (RNA) and proteins.

Mesosomes

These are convoluted membranous bodies that develop by complex invaginations of the cytoplasmic membrane into the cytoplasm and are the sites of cross wall formation in Gram-positive bacteria. They are also the principal sites of respiratory enzymes in bacteria.

Inclusions

They are sources of stored energy in bacterial cells.

Nucleus

Bacteria do not possess a well-defined nucleus and it is referred to as nuclear apparatus or nucleoid. The bacterial deoxyribonucleic acid (DNA) is not distinguishable as a clear strand and lie as a nuclear mass in the center of cytoplasm. The DNA of bacteria is haploid and replicates by binary fission. Sometimes a smaller extrachromosomal piece of DNA may be present in addition to nucleoid called plasmid.

Spores

Bacterial spores are highly resistant, dormant structures without metabolic activity and are formed in response to adverse environmental conditions. They help in the survival of the organisms during adverse environmental conditions. They do not have a role in reproduction **(Figure 3.4)**. The actual

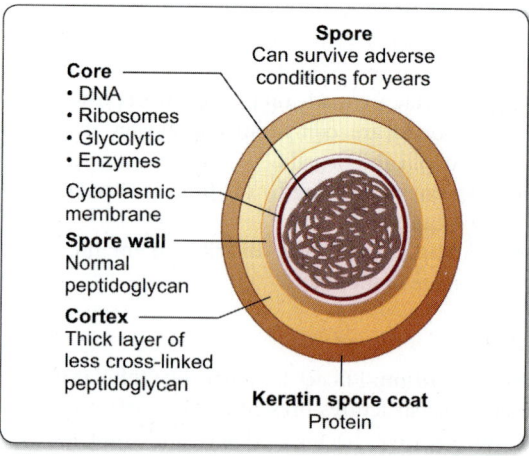

Figure 3.4: Bacterial spore

living cell, called the vegetative cell, produces a protective layer (spore) around its DNA until favorable conditions return. They are highly resistant to environmental stresses. These are formed by bacterial cells in response to environmental signals that indicate a limiting factor for growth. They germinate and become vegetative cells when the environmental stress is relieved. Hence, spore-formation is a mechanism of survival rather than a mechanism of reproduction.

REPRODUCTION OF BACTERIA

Bacteria can divide very rapidly. It multiplies by binary fission and sexual reproduction is under question. Spores are formed as a means to survive unfavorable conditions only and not as a means of asexual reproduction.

Asexual Reproduction

- **Binary fission:** The asexual reproduction in bacteria occurs through binary fission and budding. During binary fission, the chromosome copies itself, forming two genetically identical copies. Then, the cell enlarges and divides into two new daughter cells **(Figure 3.5)**.
- **Budding:** Some bacteria reproduce by budding process in which small bud develops at one end of cell. This bud develops into new cell by separating from the mother cell when suitable conditions are found.

Sexual Reproduction

Bacteria cannot reproduce sexually, but they can exchange genetic information with each other. Using a pilus, two bacteria make contact with each other and exchange genetic material.

- Bacteria can exchange DNA through the processes of conjugation, transformation, or

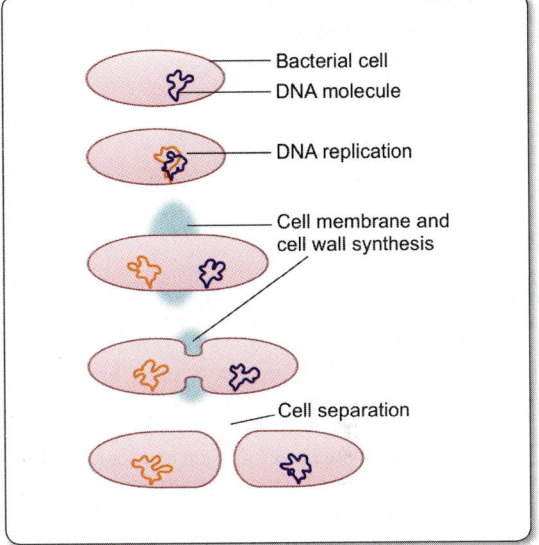

Figure 3.5: Binary fission in bacteria

transduction. But the processes are very primitive and cannot be termed as sexual reproduction.

So called sexual reproduction occurs through the following methods:

- **Conjugation:** It is a process in which the genetic material of a bacterial cell of a particular strain is transferred into that of another bacterial cell of a different strain. There is no sexual dimorphism. Of the two strains of bacteria involved, one acts as F+ donor (or male) and the other as a F- recipient (or female).
- **Transformation:** It is a physiological phenomenon by which the incorporation of DNA from one bacterium into another results in the development of a new genotype.
- **Transduction:** It is the process of transfer of DNA fragment from one bacteria to the other with the help of a bacteriophage.

Assess Yourself

LONG ANSWER QUESTION

1. How will you classify bacteria?

SHORT NOTES

1. Fimbriae
2. Spore

MULTIPLE CHOICE QUESTIONS

1. Bacterial structure involved in respiration is:
   a. Ribosome
   b. Pili
   c. Mesosome
   d. Flagella
2. Identify correct statement regarding bacteria:
   a. Respiration, cell division and sporulation are the functions of mesosome in bacteria
   b. Capsule in bacteria enables adherence to surface and protection against phagocytosis
   c. Heterotrophs are the bacteria that are unable to synthesize their own food materials
   d. All the above
3. Bacteria belongs to:
   a. Prokaryotes
   b. Eukaryotes
   c. Both
   d. None of the above
4. Site of respiration in bacteria is:
   a. Mitochondria
   b. Golgi apparatus
   c. Cell membrane
   d. Cell wall
5. Amphitrichous flagella means:
   a. Flagella all-round the cell
   b. Flagella at both ends
   c. Flagella at one end
   d. Flagella in tufts

ANSWERS TO MCQs

1. c   2. d   3. a   4. c   5. b

Methods for Study of Microbes, Culture and Isolation of Microbes

INTRODUCTION

The five basic techniques to grow, examine and characterize microorganisms are: (1) Inoculation, (2) Incubation, (3) Isolation, (4) Inspection and (5) Identification

INOCULATION (PRODUCING A CULTURE)

- To culture, one introduces a tiny sample or the inoculum into a container of a nutrient medium which provides an environment to multiply
- Selection of media with specialized functions can improve later steps of isolation and identification.

Importance of Culture

- Culturing helps in isolating an organism from different sites in body normally known to be sterile.
- Culturing bacteria is also the initial step in studying its morphology and identification.
- Bacteria have to be cultured in order to obtain antigens from developing serological assays and in preparation of vaccines.

- Certain genetic studies and manipulations of the cells also need that bacteria should be cultured *in vitro*.

Important Culture Media

An artificial culture medium to provide all the nutritional components that a bacterium needs to grow. Some of the ingredients of culture media include water, agar, peptone, casein hydrolysate, meat extract, yeast extract and malt extract.

Liquid Media

These are available for use in test-tubes, bottles or flasks. In liquid medium, bacteria grow uniformly producing general turbidity.

Solid Media

Any liquid medium can be changed into solid medium by addition of certain solidifying agents. Agar-agar (simply called agar) is the most commonly used solidifying agent that is. It obtained from the cell membranes of some species of red algae such as the genera *Gelidium*. It contains agar at a concentration of 1.5–2.0% and is an.

Semisolid Media

They are prepared with agar at a concentration of 0.5% or less. They have soft custard-like consistency and are useful for the cultivation of microaerophilic bacteria or for determination of bacterial motility.

Basal Media

Basal media are those that may be used for growth (culture) of bacteria that do not need enrichment of the media. Examples: Nutrient broth, nutrient agar and peptone water. *Staphylococcus* and Enterobacteriaceae grow in these media.

Enriched Media

These are used to grow nutritionally exacting (fastidious) bacteria. Addition of extra nutrients in the form of blood, serum, egg yolk etc., to basal medium makes it enriched media. Blood agar (Figure 4.1), chocolate agar, Loeffler's serum slope, etc. are few examples of the enriched media.

Selective Media

These media favor the growth of a particular bacterium by inhibiting the growth of undesired bacteria allowing growth of desirable bacteria. MacConkey agar, Lowenstein-Jensen media, tellurite media, etc. are few examples of selective media.

Indicator (Differential) Media

An indicator is included in the medium. A particular organism causes change in the indicator is due to biochemicals released in the medium, e.g., blood, neutral red, tellurite, etc. Blood agar and MacConkey agar are examples of indicator media.

MacConkey Agar

It is most commonly used for Enterobacteriaceae (Figure 4.2). It contains agar, peptone, sodium chloride, bile salt, lactose and neutral red. It is a selective and indicator medium:

- Selective as bile salt does not inhibit the growth of Enterobactericeae but inhibits growth of many other bacteria.
- Indicator medium as the colonies of bacteria that ferment lactose take a pink color due to production of acid. Acid turns the indicator neutral red to pink. These bacteria are called 'lactose fermenter', e.g., *Escherichia coli*. Colorless colony indicates that lactose is not fermented, i.e. the bacterium is non-lactose fermenter, e.g., *Salmonella*, *Shigella* and *Vibrio*.

Transport Media

Clinical specimens must be transported to the laboratory immediately after collection to prevent

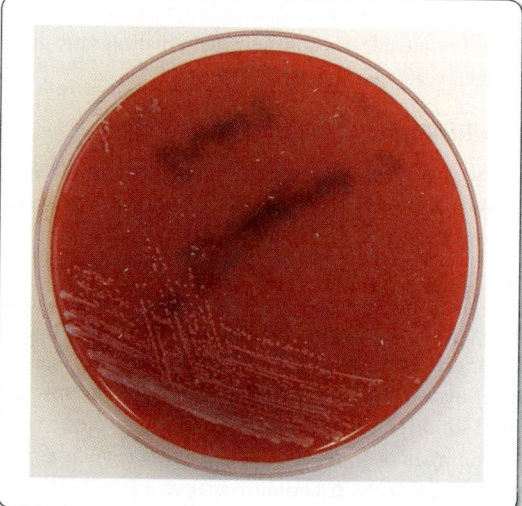

Figure 4.1: Blood agar

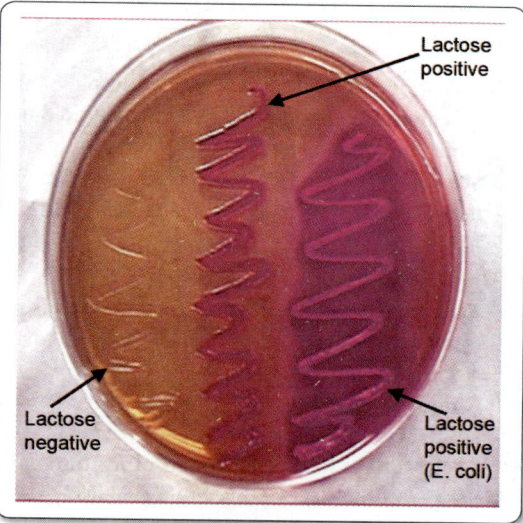

Lactose positive

Lactose negative

Lactose positive (E. coli)

Figure 4.2: MacConkey agar

overgrowth of contaminating organisms or commensals. This can be achieved by using transport media. Such media prevent drying (desiccation) of specimen, maintain the pathogen to commensal ratio and inhibit overgrowth of unwanted bacteria. Cary Blair medium and Venkatraman Ramakrishnan media are used to transport feces from suspected cholera patients.

Anaerobic Media

It is required to grow anaerobic bacteria, which needs reduced oxidation–reduction potential and extra nutrients. Such media may be reduced by physical or chemical means. Boiling the medium serves to expel any dissolved oxygen. Addition of 1% glucose, 0.1% thioglycollate, 0.1% ascorbic acid, 0.05% cysteine or red hot iron filings can reduce a medium. Robertson Cooked Meat (RCM) medium is commonly used to grow *Clostridium* species contains a 2.5 cm column of bullock heart meat and 15 mL of nutrient broth. Thioglycollate broth contains sodium thioglycollate, glucose, cysteine, yeast extract and casein hydrolysate. The organism to be cultured is kept in an anaerobic jar so that the required organism could grow in oxygen free environment **(Figure 4.3)**.

INCUBATION

- To adjust proper growth conditions of a sample
- To promote multiplication of the microbes over a period of hours, days and even weeks.
- Produces a culture—the visible growth of the microbe in the medium.

ISOLATION

The **end result** of inoculation and incubation in macroscopic forms.

The isolated microbes may take the form of separate colonies on solid media, or turbidity in broths.

Methods for Isolating Bacteria

Streak method: A small droplet of culture or sample is spread over the surface of the medium according to a pattern that gradually thins out the sample and separates the cells.

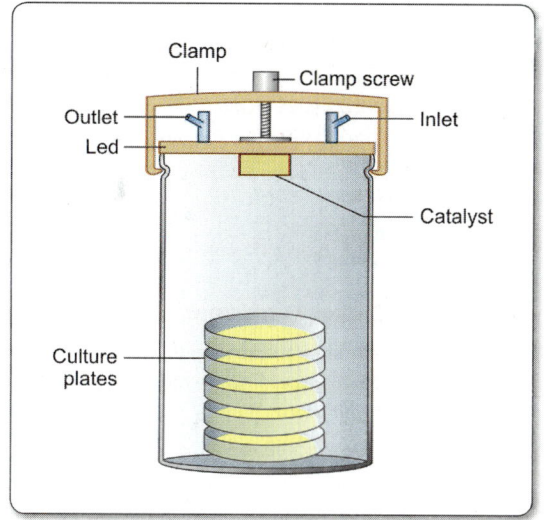

Figure 4.3: Anaerobic jar

- **Loop dilution/pour plate:** The sample is inoculated serially into a series of cooled but still liquid agar tubes so as to dilute the number of cells in each successive tube in the series. Inoculated tubes are then plated out into sterile plates and are allowed to solidify - ample space to grow as separate colonies.
- **Spread plate technique:** A small volume of liquid diluted sample is pipetted onto the surface of the medium and spread around evenly by a sterile tool (like a hockey stick). Like the streak method, cells are pushed into separate areas on the surface so that they can form individual colonies.

INSPECTION

Cultures are observed macroscopically for obvious growth characteristics (color, texture, size) that could be useful in analyzing specimen's contents.

Slides are made to assess microscopic details such as shapes, size, and motility.

Staining techniques may be used to gather specific information on microscopic morphology.

IDENTIFICATION

Specialized tests to identify microorganisms include biochemical tests to determine metabolic activities.

Assess Yourself

LONG ANSWER QUESTION

1. What is culture? Discuss various culture media.

SHORT NOTES

1. Enriched media
2. Selective media

MULTIPLE CHOICE QUESTIONS

1. Recommended transport medium for stool specimen suspected to contain *Vibrio cholerae* is:
   - a. Buffered glycerol saline medium
   - b. Venkatraman-Ramakrishanan medium
   - c. Nutrient broth
   - d. Blood agar

2. Which is an enriched media?
   - a. Selenite F broth
   - b. Peptone water
   - c. MacConkey agar
   - d. Chocolate agar

3. Agar concentration required to prepare nutrient agar is:
   - a. 1–2%
   - b. 4–6%
   - c. 0.25–0.5%
   - d. 0.5–1%

4. The media used to grow the microorganisms is known as
   - a. Culture media
   - b. Culture plate
   - c. Culture tube
   - d. All of the above

5. Most commonly used culture media for Enterobacteriaceae is:
   - a. Nutrient broth
   - b. Blood agar
   - c. Anaerobic media
   - d. MacConkey agar

6. Chocolate agar is also known as:
   - a. Loeffler's serum
   - b. Heated blood agar
   - c. Löwenstein–Jensen media
   - d. Blood agar

ANSWERS TO MCQS

1. a   **2.** b   **3.** a   **4.** a   **5.** d   **6.** b

Normal Flora of the Body

INTRODUCTION

Normal flora of the human body is a mixture of microorganisms regularly found at any anatomical site on/within the body of a healthy person. The skin and mucous membranes always harbor a variety of microorganisms that can be arranged in two groups:

- The **resident flora** consists of relatively fixed types of microorganisms regularly found in a given area at a given age; if disturbed, it promptly reestablishes itself. These are pathogenic (disease – causing) if the normal environment is disturbed or they inhabit any other site on the body.
- The **transient flora** consists of nonpathogenic or potentially pathogenic microorganisms that inhabit the skin or mucous membranes for hours, days, or week. It is derived from the environment, does not produce disease, and does not establish itself permanently on the surface.

The common sites of finding normal bacterial flora are:

- Skin
- Conjunctiva
- Nasopharynx
- Oral cavity
- Gastrointestinal tract and rectum
- Urogenital tract.

NORMAL FLORA OF THE SKIN

Skin is constantly exposed to and is in contact with the environment, the skin is particularly apt to contain transient microorganisms. The predominant resident microorganisms of the skin are aerobic and anaerobic diphtheroid bacilli (e.g., *Corynebacterium*, *Propionibacterium*); nonhemolytic aerobic and anaerobic staphylococci (*Staphylococcus epidermidis*, occasionally *S. aureus*, and *Peptostreptococcus* species); Gram-positive, aerobic, spore-forming bacilli that are present everywhere in air, water, and soil; α-hemolytic streptococci (viridans streptococci) and enterococci (enterococcus species); and Gram-negative coliform bacilli and *Acinetobacter*.

NORMAL FLORA OF CONJUNCTIVA

The conjunctiva is relatively free from bacteria due to the presence of lysozyme in the tears, which flushes the bacteria. Predominant organisms of the eyes are: *Moraxella*, diphtheroids, *S. epidermidis* and non-hemolytic streptococci.

NORMAL FLORA OF NASOPHARYNX

The nasopharynx is a natural habitat of the common pathogenic bacteria causing infection of the nose, throat, bronchi and lungs. The flora of nose harbors: diphtheroids, *Staphylococcus*, *Streptococcus*, *Haemophilus*, and *Moraxella lacunata*.

NORMAL FLORA OF THE MOUTH

The mouth contains micrococci, Gram-positive aerobic spore bearing bacilli, coliforms, *Proteus* and lactobacilli. The gums, pockets between the teeth and crypts of the tonsils have a wide spectrum of anaerobic flora like fusiform bacilli, treponemes, lactobacilli, etc. *Candida* is also found.

NORMAL FLORA OF GASTROINTESTINAL TRACT

The gastrointestinal tract of the fetus *in utero* is sterile. It becomes contaminated with organisms shortly after birth. In breast fed infants, the intestine contains lactobacilli, enterococci, colon bacilli and staphylococci. Lactobacilli and enterococci predominate in the duodenum and proximal ileum. The bacterial flora is similar in lower ileum, caecum and rectum. The anaerobic condition of colon is maintained by aerobic bacteria, which utilizes the free oxygen.

NORMAL FLORA OF THE GENITOURINARY TRACT

Mycobacterium smegmatis, a harmless commensal is found in the secretions (smegma) of both males and females genitalia. They may pose the confusion with the tubercle bacilli. Strains of *Mycoplasma* and *Ureaplasma* are frequently present as part of normal flora. *Gardnerella vaginalis*, bacteroides and alpha streptococci have been found in penile urethra. Female urethra is either sterile or contains *Staphylococcus epidermidis*. Döderlien bacilli remain in the vagina till menopause. After menopause, flora resembles that before puberty.

ADVANTAGES OF NORMAL FLORA

- They prevent or suppress the entry of the pathogens.
- These synthesize the vitamins especially vitamin K and several B group vitamins.
- The normal flora evokes the antibodies production. These antibodies cross react with pathogens having related or shared antigens, thus raising the immune status of the host against the invading pathogen.
- Colonies produced by some organisms of normal flora have a harmful effect on the pathogens.
- Endotoxins liberated by normal flora may help the defense mechanism of the body.

Assess Yourself

LONG ANSWER QUESTION

1. What is normal flora? What are its advantages?

MULTIPLE CHOICE QUESTIONS

1. All of the following are normal flora of skin, except:
a. *Corynebacterium*
b. *Moraxella*
c. *Staphylococcus*
d. *Acinetobacter*

2. Ureaplasma is frequently found as normal flora of:
a. Genitourinary tract
b. Nasopharynx
c. Gastrointestinal tract
d. Skin

3. The vitamin that is synthesized by normal flora in the body:
a. Vitamin A
b. Vitamin C
c. Vitamin K
d. Vitamin E

4. Bacteria that predominate duodenum is:
a. Lactobacilli
b. *Staphylococcus*
c. *Streptococcus*
d. *Moraxella*

5. Which bacteria is present in penile urethra?
a. *Staphylococcus epidermidis*
b. *Mycobacterium smegmatis*
c. Döderlein bacilli
d. *Gardnerella vaginalis*

ANSWERS TO MCQS

1. b   **2.** a   **3.** c   **4.** a   **5.** d

Section II • *Microorganisms*

27

Common Bacterial Diseases

INTRODUCTION

The science of study of bacteria is called bacteriology. Bacteria are the primary source of infections and diseases in human beings. Bacteria live in every climate and location on earth. Some are airborne, while others live in water or soil. A bacterial infection is a proliferation of a harmful strain of bacteria on or inside the body. Bacteria can infect any area of the body. Bacteria may also be classified as Gram-positive or Gram-negative based on the Gram staining. Gram-positive bacteria have a thick cell wall, while Gram-negative bacteria do not. Gram staining, bacterial culture with antibiotic sensitivity determination and other tests are used to identify bacterial strains and help determine the appropriate course of treatment. Let's discuss the most common disease causing bacteria.

PATHOGENIC AND NONPATHOGENIC MICROBES

Pathogenic organism: A pathogenic organism is an organism which is capable of causing diseases in a host

Nonpathogenic: Organism which do not cause diseases are called nonpathogenic

The differences between pathogenic and non-pathogenic microorganisms are given as follows in **Table 6.1**.

TABLE 6.1: Differences between Pathogenic and Nonpathogenic Bacteria

Pathogenic bacteria	Nonpathogenic bacteria
Bacteria that can cause diseases	Bacteria that do not cause disease, harm or death to another organism
Parasites	Commensals
Harmful	May be useful
Virulence genes are present in the genome	Do not possess virulence genes
Adhere to the cells of the tissues in order to escape from the fluid flows inside the body	Do not adhere to the tissue
Invades the cells of the body	Live outside the body cells
Resist phagocytosis by using a slick capsule, leucocidins, and other antiphagocytic mechanisms	Subjected to phagocytosis
Produce toxins that can alter the metabolism of the host cells	Do not produce toxins
Produce their colonies within the tissues	Do not produce colonies

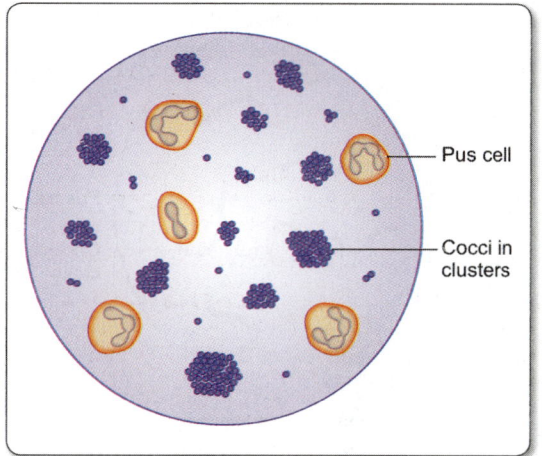

Figure 6.1: Staphylococci and pus cells

S. aureus expresses many potential virulence factors:
- Surface proteins that promote colonization of host tissues
- Factors that probably inhibit phagocytosis (capsule, immunoglobulin binding protein A)
- Toxins that damage host tissues and cause disease symptoms.

STREPTOCOCCUS

Streptococci are Gram-positive, nonmotile, nonspore-forming, catalase-negative cocci that occur in pairs or chains **(Figure 6.2)**. Older cultures may lose their Gram-positive character. Most streptococci are facultative anaerobes, and some are obligate (strict) anaerobes. Most require enriched media (blood agar). Group A streptococci have a hyaluronic acid capsule. They are aerobes but most of the species are facultative anaerobes. It requires nutrients to grow therefore, the organism grows well in an enriched medium having blood or serum as a source of extra nourishment.

STAPHYLOCOCCUS

These are Gram-positve cocci. They are spherical in shape and measure 1 μm in diameter. They are arranged in grape-like clusters **(Figure 6.1)**. Approximately, 20 species from 33 known species of *Staphylococcus* are known to cause infections in humans. The other *Staphylococcus* that is harmless commensal living in the nostrils and mouth and on skin is *S. albus*. These are nonsporing, nonmotile and noncapsulated.

Section II • Microorganisms

29

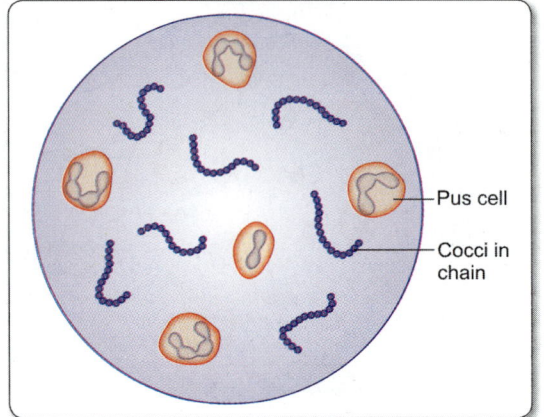

Figure 6.2: Streptococci in Gram-stained smear of pus

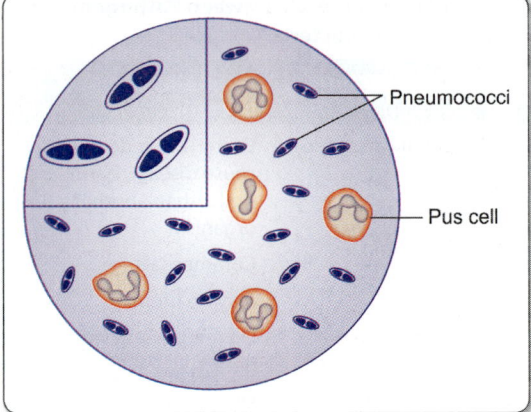

Figure 6.3: *Streptococcus pneumoniae* in pus. Inset: enlarged view

Streptococcus pneumoniae

Streptococcus pneumoniae or pneumococci are lancet-shaped, catalase-negative, capsule-forming, α-hemolytic cocci or diplococci. Autolysis is enhanced by adding bile salts **(Figure 6.3)**. *S. pneumoniae* is a normal member of the respiratory tract flora; invasion results in pneumonia. The best defined virulence factor is the polysaccharide capsule, which protects the bacterium against phagocytosis.

NEISSERIA

The genus *Neisseria* contains two important human pathogens, *N. gonorrhoeae* and *N. meningitidis*. *N. gonorrhoeae* causes gonorrhea, and *N. meningitidis* is the cause of meningococcal meningitis. *N. gonorrhoeae* is often referred to as the "gonococcus", while *N. meningitidis* is known as the "meningococcus". *N. gonorrhoeae* is a Gram-negative coccus, 0.6–1.0 μm in diameter, usually seen in pairs with adjacent flattened sides. The organism is frequently found intracellularly in polymorphonuclear leukocytes (neutrophils) of the gonorrhea pustular exudate. *N. meningitidis* is a fastidious, encapsulated, aerobic Gram-negative diplococcus **(Figure 6.4)**.

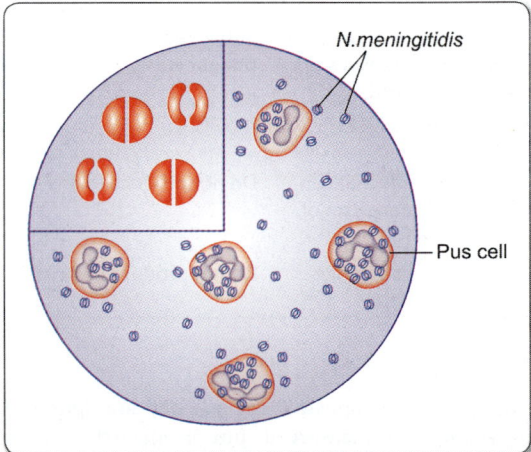

Figure 6.4: *Neisseria meningitidis* in cerebrospinal fluid. Inset: enlarged view showing adjacent sides flattened or concave and long axes parallel

CORYNEBACTERIUM DIPHTHERIAE

Corynebacterium diphtheriae is a nonmotile, noncapsulated, club-shaped, Gram-positive bacillus **(Figure 6.5)**. *C. diphtheriae* spreads by droplets, secretions, or direct contact. It causes diphtheria in

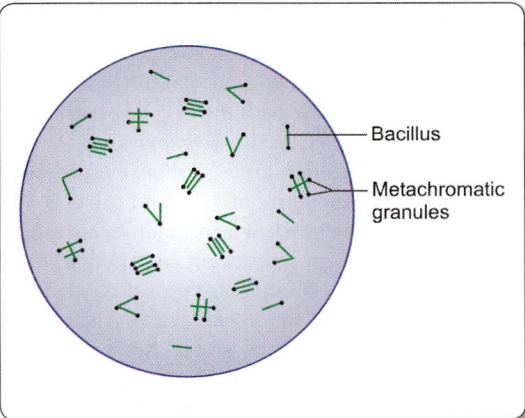

Figure 6.5: *Corynebacterium diphtheriae* showing metachromatic granules and Chinese letter arrangement

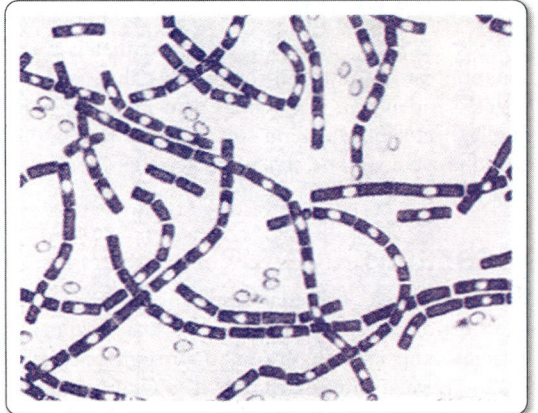

Figure 6.6: Bacillus anthracis

humans when toxin is produced with the help of a particular bacteriophage – β phage, which provides it with toxin producing gene. This is known as phage conversion. When the bacteria are cured of phage, toxigenicity is lost.

CHLAMYDIAE TRACHOMATIS

Amydiae are small Gram-negative obligate intracellular microorganisms that preferentially infect squamocolumnar epithelial cells. They include the genera *Chlamydia* (of which the type species is *Chlamydia trachomatis*) and *Chlamydophila* (e.g., *Chlamydophila pneumoniae* and *Chlamydophila psittaci*). They lack peptidoglycan in cell wall and cannot produce ATP on their own, so they use host's energy – energy parasites.

BACILLUS ANTHRACIS

These are Gram-positive spore bearing rods. They are nonmotile and arranged in chains which is surrounded by capsule. They appear as bamboo sticks under microscope **(Figure 6.6)**. The spores can survive in soil for very long period of time. They are aerobes and facultative anaerobes. On nutrient agar, colonies appear as greyish white, round and irregularly raised. Under low power microscope, the edges of colonies appear as tangled mass of hairy curls—called medusa head.

CLOSTRIDIUM TETANI

Clostridium is the genus of rod-shaped, usually Gram-positive bacteria, members of which are found in soil, water, and the intestinal tracts of humans and other animals. Most species grow only in the complete absence of oxygen. Dormant cells are highly resistant to heat, desiccation, and toxic chemicals and detergents. It is Gram-positive in young cultures, but becomes Gram-negative upon sporulation.

VIBRIO CHOLERAE

Vibrio cholerae is a "comma"-shaped Gram-negative bacteria with a single, polar flagellum for movement. There are numerous strains of *V. cholerae*, some of which are pathogenic and some of which are not. They live in mutual association with marine life. *Vibrio cholerae* is one of the important members of this genus, which causes cholera in humans. They are aerobes and facultative anaerobes. It does not require enriched media to grow (not fastidious) and grow at an optimum temperature of 37°C. It produces moist, translucent and round colonies when inoculated on nutrient agar with bluish tinge in transmitted light.

YERSINIA PESTIS

Yersinia pestis is a zoonotic pathogen that is most commonly transmitted through fleas that feed on infected rodents. *Y. pestis* is a Gram-negative, non-motile, non-spore-forming coccobacillus that is also a facultative anaerobe. They are generally arranged singly in short chains or in small groups.

ESCHERICHIA COLI

Escherichia coli bacteria normally live in the intestines of people and animals. Most *E. coli* are harmless and actually are an important part of a healthy human intestinal tract. It is Gram-negative bacillus. The organism is non-capsulated and $1–3 \times 0.4–0.7\ \mu m$ in size. Most of the strains are motile due to peritrichous flagella. Fimbriae and capsules are present on majority of the strains. However, some *E. coli* are pathogenic; they can cause illness, either diarrhea or illness outside of the intestinal tract. The types of *E. coli* that can cause diarrhea can be transmitted through contaminated water or food, or through contact with animals or persons.

E. coli consists of a diverse group of bacteria. Pathogenic *E. coli* strains are categorized into pathotypes. Six pathotypes are associated with diarrhea and collectively are referred to as diarrheagenic *E. coli*.

KLEBSIELLA

Klebsiella bacteria are normally found in the human intestines (where they do not cause disease). They are also found in human stool (feces). *Klebsiella* is a type of Gram-negative, facultative anaerobic, nonmotile bacteria that can cause different types of healthcare-associated infections, including pneumonia, bloodstream infections, wound or surgical site infections and meningitis.

SALMONELLA TYPHI

These are Gram-negative, non-capsulated, non-sporing bacilli, which are $2–4\ \mu m \times 0.6\ \mu m$ in size. Most of the strains are motile with the help of peritrichous flagella except *S. pullorum* and *S. gallinarum*.

These are aerobes and facultative anaerobes that grow at a temperature of 37°C and pH 6–8. On ordinary media like nutrient agar, colonies are moist, greyish-white, convex, translucent and circular.

S. typhi is the causative agent of typhoid fever or enteric fever. *S. paratyphi* causes disease of less severity. The bacteria enters the body with contaminated water or food. Incubation period is 10–14 days. The bacteria attach themselves to the microvilli and invades the small intestine.

SHIGELLA

Shigella is a group of organisms that are *Gram-negative aerobes or facultative anaerobes*. The organism is non-flagellate, noncapsulated, nonsporing and nonmotile bacillus. It measures about $2–4\ \mu m \times 0.6\ \mu m$ in size.

Shigellosis is an *acute diarrheal disease* caused by *Shigella* and is one of the major health problems in developing countries with poor sanitation. Human beings act as natural reservoir of this organism. Infection is transmitted through contaminated food or water (feco-oral route of transmission).

MYCOBACTERIUM

The organisms included in Mycobacteria genus are nonmotile, Gram-positive and very slow growing bacilli. These are obligate parasites, opportunistic pathogens or occur as saprophytes. The genus mycobacteria can be divided into three major groups;
- *Mycobacterium tuberculosis*: Causes tuberculosis
- *Mycobacterium leprae*: Causes leprosy
- Nontuberculous mycobacteria.

COMMON BACTERIAL DISEASES (TABLE 6.2)

TABLE 6.2: Common Bacterial Diseases

Disease and pathogen	Transmission and incubation period	Symptoms	Prevention and treatment
Disease: Actinomycosis **Pathogen:** *Actinomyces*	**Transmission:** Person-to-person via contact of the oral flora **Incubation period:** From several days to several years	Commonly affects jaw. Also affects the brain, lungs or intestines The bacterium is normally present in mouth but it may become pathogenic when a tooth is extracted, causing the slow formation of abscesses and ulcers	**Treatment:** Antibiotics for several months to a year. Surgical drainage or removal of the lesion may be needed **Prevention:** Good oral hygiene and regular dentist visits prevent some forms of actinomycosis
Disease: Anthrax **Pathogen:** *Bacillus anthracis*	**Transmission:** By contact with farm animal hair, hides or excretions	In man, the disease attacks either the lungs, causing pneumonia (wool sorter's disease), or the skin, producing severe ulceration (malignant pustule)	**Treatment:** Administration of large doses of penicillin or tetracycline
Disease: Botulism (and Infant botulism) **Pathogen:** *Clostridium botulinum*	**Transmission:** Through contamination of food (food poisoning) **Incubation period:** Infants: 3–30 days **Children and adults:** 12–72 hours	**Infants:** Lethargy, weakness, poor feeding, constipation, poor head control, poor gag and sucking reflex **Children and adults:** Double vision, blurred vision, drooping eyelids, slurred speech, difficulty swallowing, dry mouth and muscle weakness	**Treatment:** Penicillin
Disease: Brucellosis **Pathogen:** *Brucella* genus	**Transmission:** By direct contact or untreated/contaminated milk of animals	Abdominal pain, back pain, chills, excessive sweating, fatigue, fever, headache, joint pain, loss of appetite, weakness, weight loss	**Treatment:** Antibiotics **Prevention:** Avoid unpasteurized dairy foods. Cook meat thoroughly. Wear gloves. Take safety precautions in high-risk workplaces. Vaccinate domestic animals

Contd...

Disease and pathogen	Transmission and incubation period	Symptoms	Prevention and treatment
Disease: Cellulitis **Pathogen:** Group A *Streptococcus* and *Staphylococcus*	**Transmission:** It may infected after any event that causes a break in the skin, such as: • Surgery • A cut or bite • A new tattoo or piercing • Skin breakdown, such as eczema, psoriasis, or a fungal infection like athlete's foot	At first, the infected area will be warm, red, swollen, and tender. If the infection spreads, one may have a fever, chills, and swollen lymph nodes	**Treatment:** Antibiotics
Disease: Chancroid **Pathogen:** *Haemophilus ducreyi*	**Transmission:** Sexual contact with an infected person **Incubation period:** 1–2 weeks	Chancroid begins with a small bump that becomes an ulcer within a day of its appearance. The ulcer characteristically: • Ranges in size dramatically from 3 to 50 mm (1/8 inch to two inches) across is painful • Has sharply defined, undermined borders • Has irregular or ragged borders • Has a base that is covered with a grey or yellowish-grey material • Has a base that bleeds easily, if traumatized or scraped painful lymphadeno-pathy occurs in 30–60% of patients	**Treatment:** The CDC recommendation for chancroid is a single oral dose (1 g) of Azithromycin or a single IM dose of Ceftriaxone or oral Erythromycin for 7 days. **Prevention:** Avoid all forms of sexual activity with infected persons
Disease: Chlamydia (Chlamydiasis) **Pathogen:** *Chlamydia trachomatis*	**Transmission:** By vaginal, anal, or oral sex. It can also be passed from an infected mother to her baby during vaginal childbirth	**In women:** Abnormal vaginal discharge that may have an odor. Bleeding between periods. Painful periods. Abdominal pain with fever. Pain while having sex. Itching or burning in or around the vagina. Pain when urinating. **In men:** Small amounts of clear or cloudy discharge from the tip of the penis. Painful urination. Burning and itching around the opening of the penis. Pain and swelling around the testicles.	**Treatment:** Antibiotics

Contd...

Contd...

Disease and pathogen	Transmission and incubation period	Symptoms	Prevention and treatment
Disease: Cholera **Pathogen:** *Vibrio cholerae (Vibrio comma)*	**Transmission:** Through contaminated food and water. **Incubation period:** 6 hours to 3 days	Severe diarrhea, irritation of skin around anus, rice water stool; vomiting and muscular cramps, dehydration of the body	Anti- or Bilivaccine
Disease: *Clostridium* infection (food poisoning) **Pathogen:** *Clostridium perfringens*	**Transmission:** Beef, poultry, gravies **Incubation period:** 6–24 hours	Diarrhea and abdominal cramps (not fever or vomiting)	• Thoroughly cook foods to a safe internal temperature • Use a food thermometer • Keep food hot after cooking • Refrigerate perishable foods within two hours (at 40°F or below)
Disease: Diphtheria **Pathogen:** *Corynebacterium diphtheriae*	**Transmission:** Attacks children from 1 to 5 years of age **Incubation period:** 2–4 days	Upper respiratory tract illness having sore throat, an adherent layer on the tonsils, nasal cavity and pharynx. Toxins produce high fever, damage the nervous system and heart	**Prevention:** By active immunization; DT or DPT (bivalent or trivalent) at the age of 3–12 months; 3 doses at the interval of 4–6 weeks.
Disease: Epidemic typhus **Pathogen:** *Rickettsia prowazekii*	**Transmission:** Feeding on a human who carries the bacillus infects the louse. *R. prowazekii* grows in the louse's gut and is excreted in its feces. The disease is then transmitted to an uninfected human who scratches the louse bite (which itches) and rubs the feces into the wound **Incubation period:** 1–2 weeks	Severe headache, a sustained high fever, cough, rash, severe muscle pain, chills, falling blood pressure, stupor, sensitivity to light, delirium and death. A rash begins on the chest about five days after the fever appears, and spreads to the trunk and extremities. A symptom common to all forms of typhus is a fever which may reach 102°F	**Treatment:** Antibiotics Intravenous fluids and oxygen may be needed to stabilize the patient
Disease: Gonorrhea **Pathogen:** *Neisseria gonorrhoeae*	**Transmission:** Through sexual contact (venereal disease)	Burning and pain during micturition. Leads to sterility	**Treatment:** Antibiotics like penicillin G

Disease and pathogen	Transmission and incubation period	Symptoms	Prevention and treatment
Disease: Leprosy (Hansen's disease) **Pathogen:** *Mycobacterium leprae*	**Transmission:** By direct contact with infected person **Incubation period:** 1–5 years	Granulomatous disease of the peripheral nerves and mucosa of the upper respiratory tract. Ulcers, nodules, scab deformities of fingers and toes, in particular nerves are being infected	**Treatment:** Lepromin skin test confirms the presence of the disease **Drugs:** Dapsone (DDS; 4, 4' diaminodiphenyl-sulfone) given for several years
Disease: Leptospirosis **Pathogen:** *Leptospira* genus	**Transmission:** Through rodents etc. It is often transmitted by animal urine or water containing animal urine. **Incubation period:** 4–14 day	High fever, severe headache, chills, muscle aches, and vomiting, and may include jaundice, red eyes, abdominal pain, diarrhea, and rash. Initial presentation may resemble pneumonia Biphasic disease with meningitis, liver damage and renal failure	
Disease: Meningitis (Bacterial) **Pathogen:** *Neisseria meningitidis*	**Transmission:** It usually occurs when bacteria enter the bloodstream and migrate to the brain and spinal cord. But it can also occur when bacteria directly invade the meninges, as a result of an ear or sinus infection, or a skull fracture, or rarely, after some surgeries	• Sudden high fever • Severe headache that isn't easily confused with other types of headache • Stiff neck • Vomiting or nausea with headache • Confusion or difficulty concentrating • Seizures • Sleepiness or difficulty waking up • Sensitivity to light • Lack of interest in drinking and eating • Skin rash in some cases, such as in meningococcal meningitis • Signs in newborns • High fever • Constant crying • Excessive sleepiness or irritability • Inactivity or sluggishness • Poor feeding • A bulge in the soft spot on top of a baby's head (fontanel) • Stiffness in a baby's body and neck	**Treatment:** • Intravenous antibiotics • Cortisone medications

Contd...

Disease and pathogen	Transmission and incubation period	Symptoms	Prevention and treatment
Disease: Mycoplasma pneumonia **Pathogen:** *Mycoplasma pneumoniae*	**Transmission:** From person to person	• Persistent fever • Dry cough • Malaise • Fever	**Treatment:** • Antibiotics • Corticosteroids • Immunomodulatory therapy
Disease: Plague **Pathogen:** *Yersinia (Pasteurella) pestis*	**Transmission:** By rats and other rodents. Vector is a flea, *Xenopsylla cheopsis* which feeds on infected rodents and may bite man.	Inflammation of the lymphatics, subcutaneous tissues and viscera; diffused hemorrhage into the skin.	**Treatment:** **Drugs:** Streptomycin, Chloromycin and Kanamycin
Disease: Pneumonia **Pathogen:** *Streptococcus pneumoniae*	**Transmission:** Through contact with infected person **Incubation period:** 1–3 days	Mucus collects in alveoli of the lungs. Restlessness, cough and fever	**Treatment:** Antibiotics like tetracycline or penicillin G
Disease: Scarlet fever (Scarlatina) **Pathogen:** *Streptococcus pyogenes*	**Transmission:** Infection may occur through blood stream or skin and underlying tissues.	Sore throat, fever and a rash over the upper body that may spread to cover almost the entire body.	**Treatment:** Antibiotics
Disease: Shigellosis (Bacillary dysentery) **Pathogen:** *Shigella* genus	**Transmission:** • From one infected person to the next • From stool	Dysentery due to poor hygiene.	**Treatment:** Antibiotic treatment.
Disease: Syphilis **Pathogen:** *Treponema pallidum*	**Transmission:** Through sexual contact. Also caused by kissing and using clothing of infected persons. **Incubation period:** 15–20 days	Affects mucous membrane of genital tract, rectum and mouth	Antibiotics like penicillin G or ampicillin

Contd...

Disease and pathogen	Transmission and incubation period	Symptoms	Prevention and treatment
Disease: Tetanus (Lockjaw) **Pathogen:** *Clostridium tetani* (Gram +ve)	**Transmission:** CNS of man contaminated with dust, soil or water. **Incubation period:** 5–12 years	Toxin, tetanospasmin affects nervous system. Painful stiffness of the neck (lock jaw) and difficulty in swallowing; sensitivity to noise, fever. Prolonged contraction of skeletal muscle fibers	**Prevention:** Anti-tetanus (tetanal immune globulin) injection or vaccination in childhood with tetanus toxoid.
Disease: Trachoma **Pathogen:** *Chlamydia trachomatis*	**Transmission:** By direct contact or using infective cloths of a patient. **Incubation period:** 5–10 days	Inflammation of cornea, redness of eye and discomfort and pain. Probably leading to blindness	Tetracycline and erythromycin as ophthalmic ointments
Disease: Tuberculosis **Pathogen:** *Mycobacterium tuberculosis*	**Transmission:** By contact, i.e. coughing, sneezing, spitting, talking etc. **Incubation period:** 2 weeks	Generally attacks the lungs but may affect central nervous system, circulatory system, lymphatic system, bones, joints, genitourinary system and skin. Bacteria release toxin-tuberculin, results in fever. Lungs are affected. Weakness and loss of weight.	Streptomycin and para-amino salicylic acid (PAS) or BCG vaccination
Disease: Typhoid fever **Pathogen:** *Salmonella typhi*	**Transmission:** Ingestion of food or water adulterated with feces of an infected person. **Incubation period:** 4 weeks	Continuous fever, headache and lethargy. It is followed by enlargement of spleen, pain in stomach and rose coloured rashes on body.	**Drug:** Chloramphenicol; inoculation is given every year.

Color Plates of Bacterial Diseases

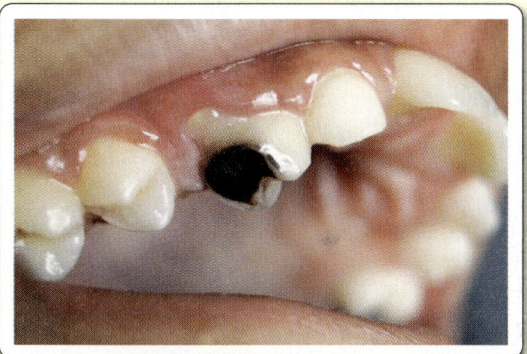

Color plate 1: Dental caries

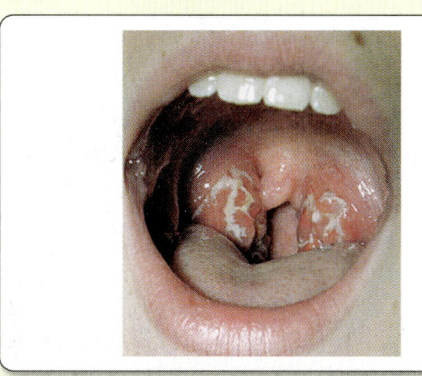

Color plate 2: Streptococcal pharyngitis

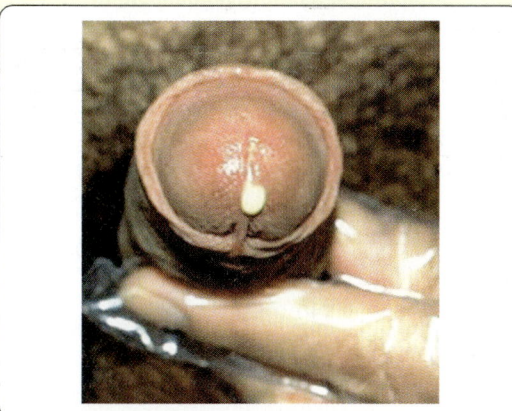

Color plate 3: Gonorrhea

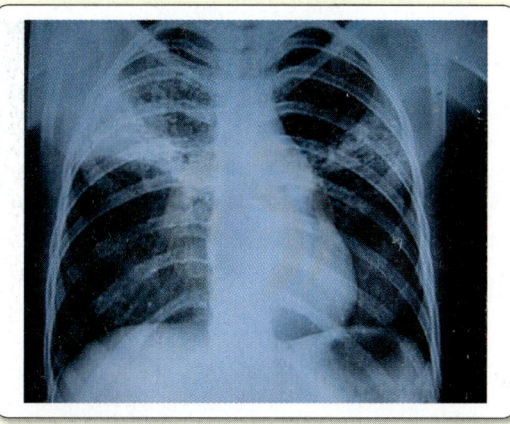

Color plate 4: Tuberculosis

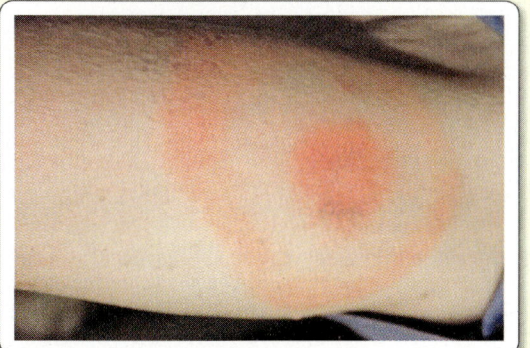

Color plate 5: Lyme Disease

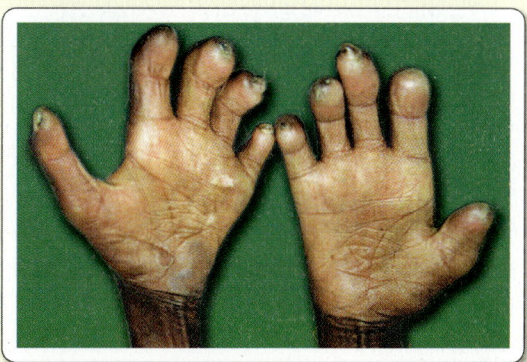

Color plate 6: Leprosy

Assess Yourself

Long Answer Questions

1. What are pathogenic and nonpathogenic bacteria.
2. Write differences between pathogenic and nonpathogenic bacteria.

Short Notes

1. Leprosy
2. Tuberculosis

Multiple Choice Questions

1. Drug of choice to treat leprosy is:
   - a. Rifampicin
   - b. Acyclovir
   - c. Zidovudine
   - d. Dapsone

2. Food poisoning is caused by:
   - a. *Clostridium perfringens*
   - b. *Clostridium botulinum*
   - c. *Corynebacterium diphtheriae*
   - d. *Clostridium tetani*

3. The causative agent of tuberculosis (TB) is:
   - a. *Mycobacterium tuberculosis*
   - b. *Mycobacterium leprae*
   - c. *Treponema pallidum*
   - d. *Borrelia* species

4. The causative agent of plague is:
   - a. Mosquito
   - b. *Yersinia pestis*
   - c. *Mycobacterium tuberculosis*
   - d. *Mycobacterium lepare*

5. Characteristic feature of *Staphylococcus aureus* is:
   - a. It is aerobic
   - b. It produces golden yellow colonies
   - c. Non-sporing
   - d. All of the above

6. Which of the following is a Gram-positive cocci?
   - a. *Streptococcus*
   - b. *Neisseria*
   - c. *Escherichia*
   - d. *Corynebacterium*

7. Who discovered Vibrio cholerae (cholera)?
   - a. Robert Koch
   - b. Ronald Ross
   - c. Filippo Pacini
   - d. Alexander Flaming

8. Who discovered the Mycobacterium leprae bacilli?
   - a. Edward Jenner
   - b. Yersin
   - c. Loeffler
   - d. Hansen

9. Presence of pathogenic bacteria in the blood is known as:
   - a. Toxemia
   - b. Septicemia
   - c. Bacteremia
   - d. All of the above

Answers to MCQs

1. d **2.** b **3.** a **4.** b **5.** d **6.** a **7.** a, c **8.** d **9.** c

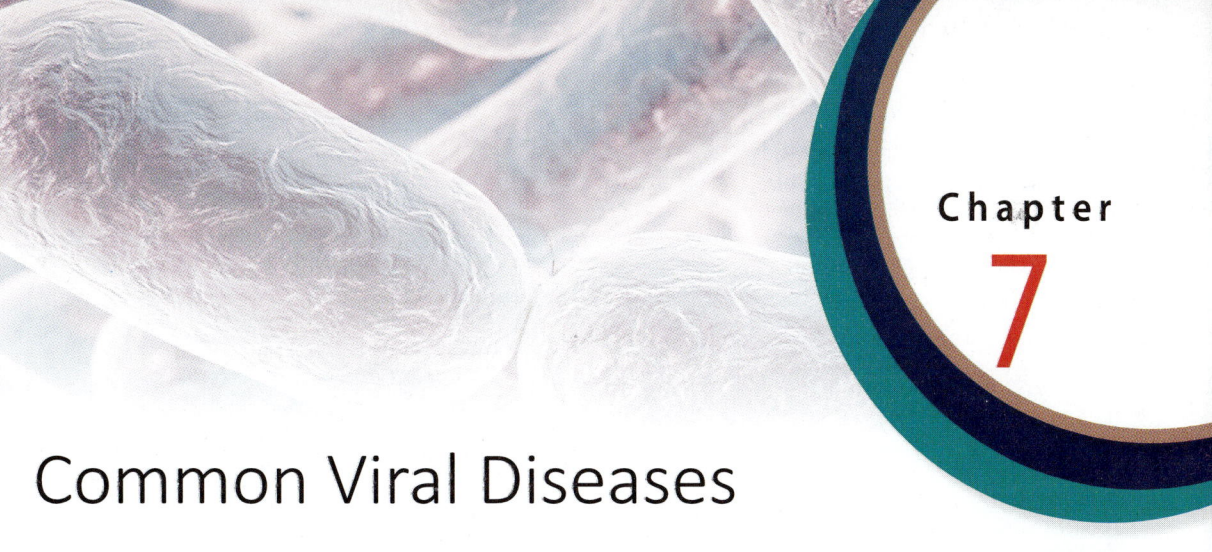

Common Viral Diseases

INTRODUCTION

Viruses are non-cellular organisms, which are made up of genetic material and protein that can invade living cells. They can only reproduce by infecting living cells. These microorganisms belong to the family viridae.

They are considered both a living and nonliving thing.

Viruses are very small and they are measured in nanometers. Their size ranges from 20 nanometers to 250 nanometers. They can only be seen with an electron microscope. They are composed of a core of deoxyribonucleic acid (DNA) or ribonucleic acid (RNA) surrounded by a protein coat.

CHARACTERISTICS OF VIRUSES

- They are noncellular.
- They do not respire, do not metabolize and do not grow but they do multiply when they are inside the host's cells.
- They contain a protein coat called the capsid.
- They have a nucleic acid core containing DNA or RNA.
- Ribosomes and enzymes are absent, which are needed for metabolism.
- They are enclosed in a protective envelope.
- They have spikes, which help them to attach to the host cell.
- They are considered both as living and nonliving things, as viruses are inactive when they are outside of host cells and are active inside of host cells and they make use of raw materials and enzymes of the host cell to multiply and cause several infections.

STRUCTURE OF VIRUSES

Because most viruses are extremely well adapted to their host organism, virus structure varies greatly. However, there are some general structural characteristics that all viruses share.

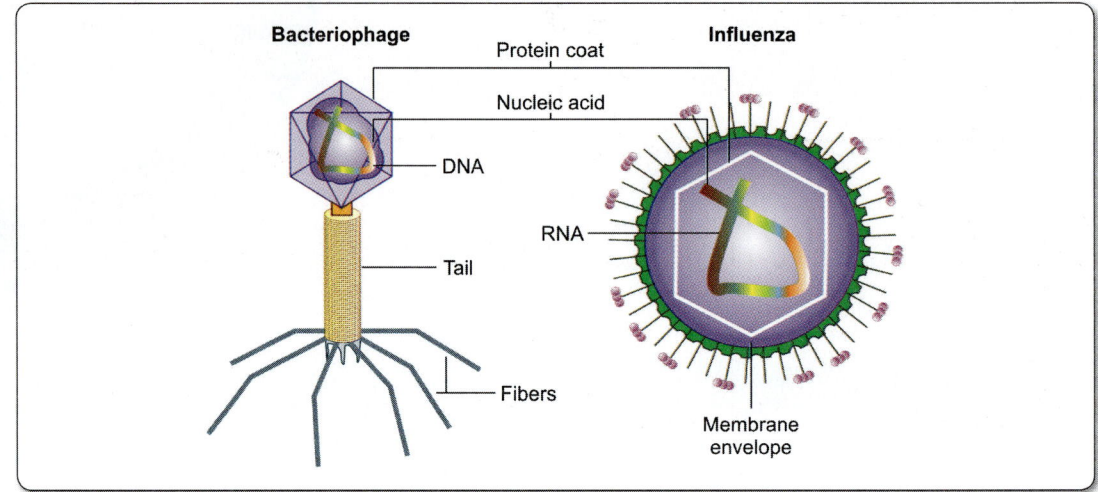

Figure 7.1: Structure of viruses

A fully assembled infectious virus is called a virion. The simplest virions consist of two basic components: nucleic acid (single- or double-stranded RNA or DNA) and a protein coat, the capsid, which functions as a shell to protect the viral genome from nucleases and which during infection attaches the virion to specific receptors exposed on the prospective host cell. Capsid proteins are coded for by the virus genome.

Capsids are formed as single or double protein shells and consist of only one or a few structural protein species. Therefore, multiple protein copies must self-assemble to form the continuous three-dimensional capsid structure **(Figure 7.1)**.

Some virus families have an additional covering, called the envelope, which is usually derived in part from modified host cell membranes. This viral envelope consist of a lipid bilayer that closely surrounds a shell of virus-encoded membrane-associated proteins.

POX VIRUSES

The poxviruses are large enough to be seen under light microscope. The virus is brick shaped under the electron microscope but it could be an artefact as it appears as spherical or ovoid in thin sections of infected tissues with a disc-like nucleoid **(Figure 7.2)**. Poxviruses exist throughout the world and cause

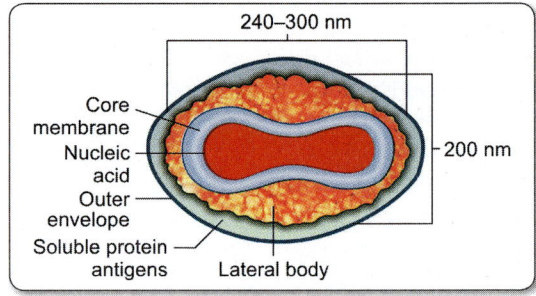

Figure 7.2: Structure of pox virus

disease in humans and many other types of animals. Poxvirus infections typically result in the formation of lesions, skin nodules, or disseminated rash.

Infection in humans usually occurs due to contact with contaminated animals, people, or materials. While some poxviruses, such as smallpox (variola virus), no longer exist in nature, other poxviruses can still cause disease. These include monkeypox virus, orf virus, molluscum contagiosum, and others.

HERPES VIRUS

Hepesviruses are icosahederal with double-stranded DNA and covered with lipid envelop. The capsid is made up of 162 capsomers **(Figure 7.3)**. The envelope is derived from the host cell membrane through

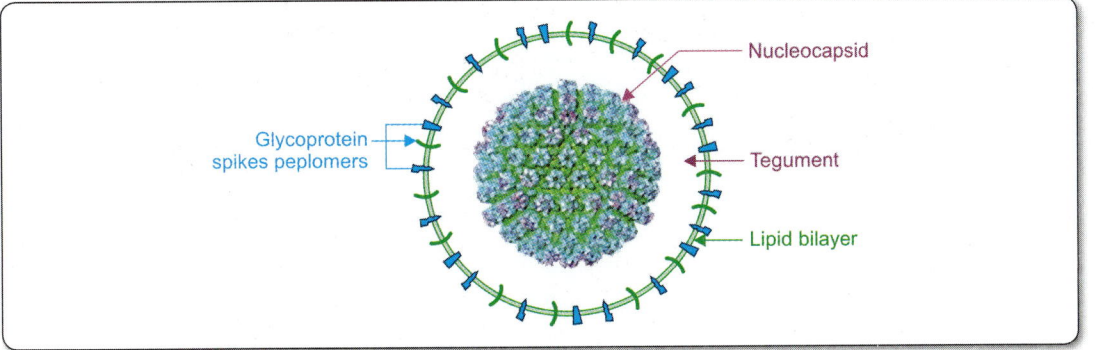

Figure 7.3: Herpes virus

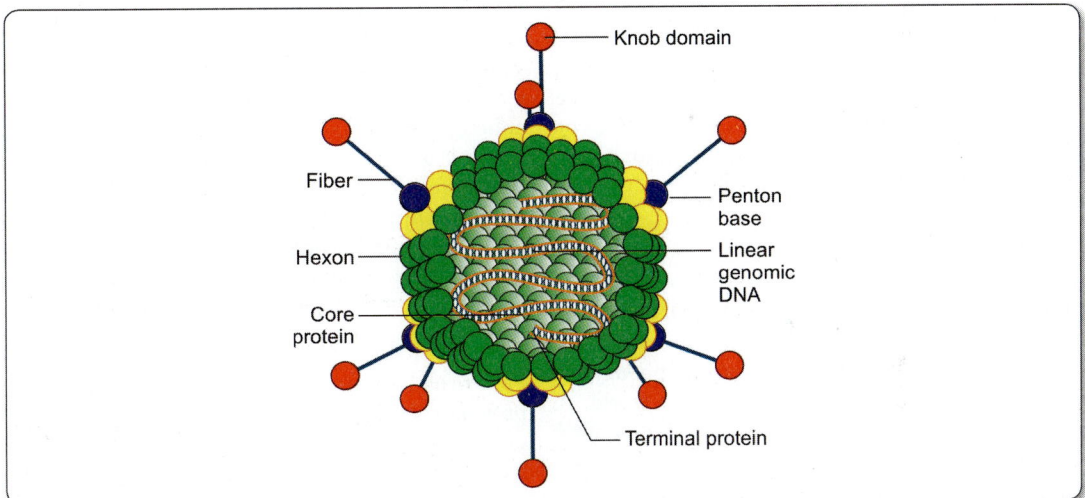

Figure 7.4: Adenovirus

which virion buds out in replication phase. Envelope carries surface spikes – about 8 nm in length. They are of two types: herpes simplex virus type 1 (HSV-1) and type 2 (HSV-2). Both are closely related but differ in epidemiology. HSV-1 is traditionally associated with orofacial disease, while HSV-2 is traditionally associated with genital disease.

ADENOVIRUS

Adenovirus, a DNA virus, was first isolated in the 1950s in adenoid tissue–derived cell cultures, hence the name. These primary cell cultures were often noted to spontaneously degenerate over time, and adenoviruses are now known to be a common cause of asymptomatic respiratory tract infection that produces *in vitro* cytolysis in these tissues. The virus is capable of infecting multiple organ systems; however, most infections are asymptomatic. Adenovirus is often cultured from the pharynx and stool of asymptomatic children **(Figure 7.4)**.

HEPATITIS VIRUSES

The hepatitis viruses include a range of unrelated and often highly unusual human pathogens.

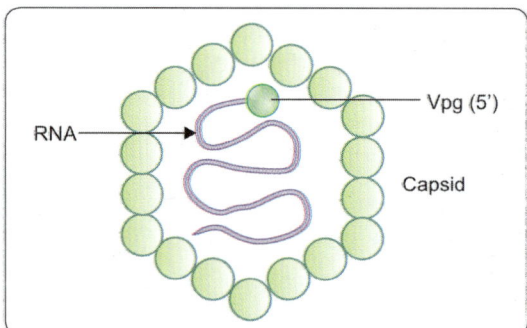

Figure 7.5: Hepatitis A virus

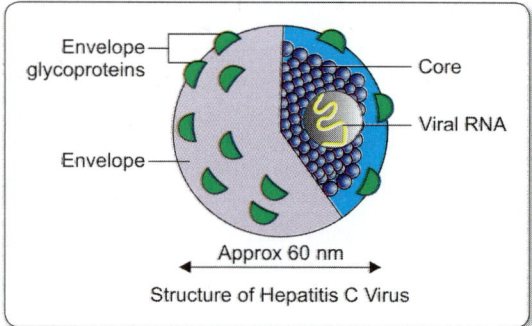

Figure 7.7: Hepatitis C virus

Hepatitis A Virus

Hepatitis A virus (HAV), classified as hepatovirus, is a small, unenveloped symmetrical RNA virus, which shares many of the characteristics of the picornavirus family, and is the cause of infectious or epidemic hepatitis transmitted by the fecal-oral route **(Figure 7.5)**.

Hepatitis B Virus

Hepatitis B virus (HBV), a member of the hepadnavirus group, double-stranded DNA viruses which replicates, unusually, by reverse transcription. Hepatitis B virus is endemic in the human population and hyperendemic in many parts of the world. A number of variants of this virus have been described **(Figure 7.6)**.

Hepatitis C Virus

Hepatitis C virus (HCV), is an enveloped single-stranded RNA virus, which appears to be distantly related (possibly in its evolution) to flaviviruses, although hepatitis C is not transmitted by arthropod vectors. Several genotypes have been identified. Infection with this more recently identified virus is common in many countries. Hepatitis C virus is associated with chronic liver disease and also with primary liver cancer in some countries **(Figure 7.7)**.

POLIO VIRUS

Poliovirus is composed of an RNA genome and a protein capsid. The genome is a single-stranded positive-sense RNA genome that is about 7500 nucleotides long. The viral particle is about 30 nm

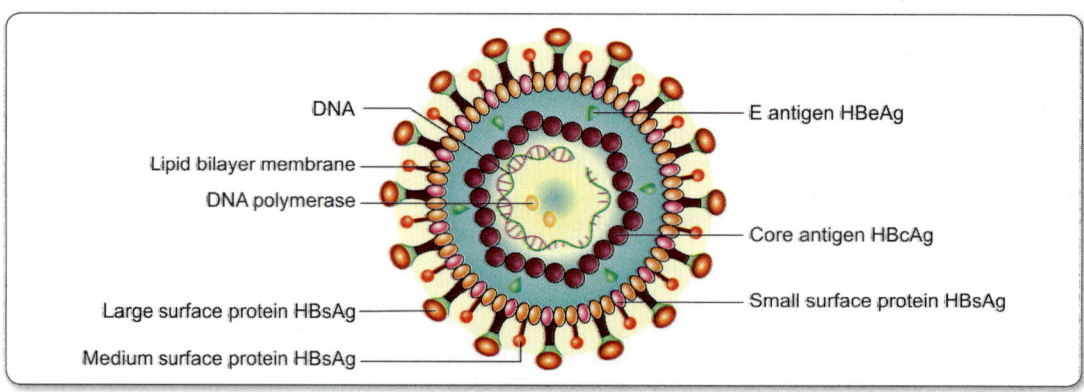

Figure 7.6: Hepatitis B virus

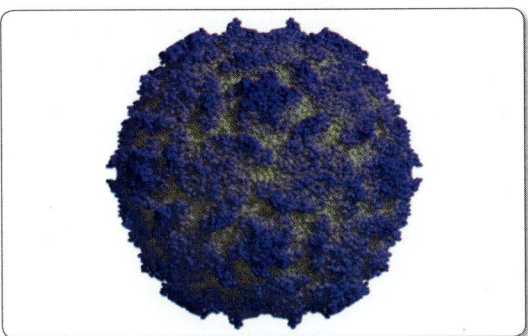

Figure 7.8: Polio virus

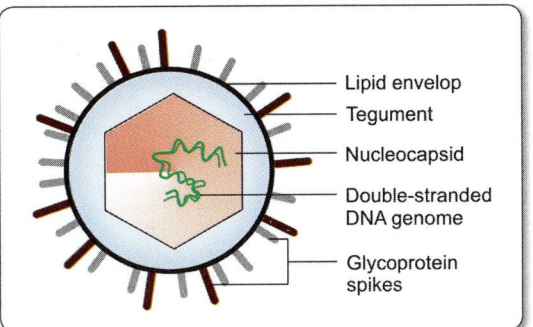

Figure 7.9: Varicella zoster virus

in diameter with icosahedral symmetry. Because of its short genome and its simple composition—only RNA and a nonenveloped icosahedral protein coat that encapsulates it, poliovirus is widely regarded as the simplest significant virus **(Figure 7.8)**.

VARICELLA ZOSTER VIRUS

Varicella zoster virus (VZV) is an exclusively human virus that belongs to the α-herpesvirus family. VZV is present worldwide and is highly infectious. Primary infection leads to acute varicella or "chicken pox", usually from exposure either through direct contact with a skin lesion or through airborne spread from respiratory droplets. After initial infection, VZV establishes lifelong latency in cranial nerve and dorsal root ganglia, and can get reactivated years to decades later as herpes zoster (HZ) or "shingles" **(Figure 7.9)**.

EPSTEIN BARR VIRUS

The virus causes diseases of lymphoid system. In 1987, EBV was isolated from clinical samples of Hodgkin's lymphoma.

The virus has also been found in people on immunosuppressive medicines after having organ transplant and is associated with post-transplant lymphoproliferative disease. There is increased number of lymphocytes in the bloodstream or B-cell lymphoma may be observed.

CYTOMEGALOVIRUS

Cytomegalovirus is a common herpes virus. Many people do not know they have it, because they may have no symptoms. But the virus, which remains dormant in the body, can cause complications during pregnancy and for people with a weakened immune system. The virus spreads through bodily fluids, and it can be passed on from a pregnant mother to her unborn baby. Also known as HCMV, CMV, or Human Herpes virus 5 (HHV-5), cytomegalovirus is most commonly transmitted to a developing fetus.

PARAMYXOVIRUSES

Mumps Virus

It is enveloped virus having single stranded RNA. Envelop is made up of lipid bilayer derived from host cell membrane. It causes mumps. The disease is highly contagious and could cause deafness in children. It is transmitted through respiratory route by droplets or accidental contact with infected saliva of a patient.

Measles Virus

Measles is one of the infectious diseases of childhood, caused by rubeola virus. The virus has single stranded RNA and is enveloped with helical symmetry. Virus lacks neuraminidases but hemagglutinins are present on envelope and serve as attachment sites to the host cells. The virus has only one serotype and is antigenically stable. It causes measles. Infection is spread by physical contact with patient suffering from disease or accidental contact with fomites infected with patient's respiratory tract secretions **(Figure 7.10)**.

45

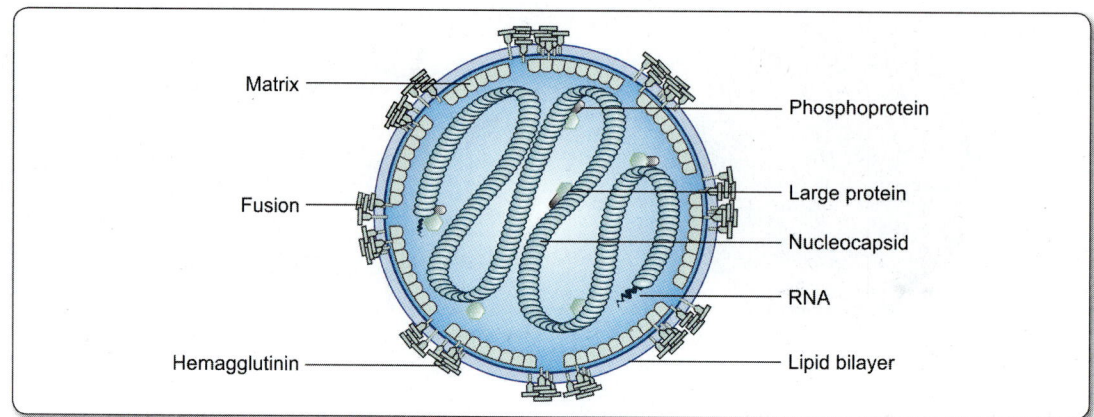

Figure 7.10: Measles virus

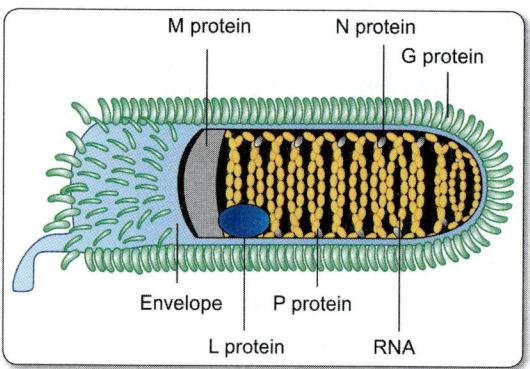

Figure 7.11: Rabies virus

Rabies Virus

Rabies is a zoonotic disease. Rabies virus is a rod- or bullet-shaped, single-stranded, negative-sense, unsegmented, enveloped RNA virus. The virus genome encodes five proteins. Rabies virus causes acute infection of the central nervous system. Five general stages are recognized in humans: incubation, prodrome, acute neurologic period, coma, and death. The incubation period is exceptionally variable, ranging from fewer than 10 days to longer than 2 years, but is usually 1–3 months **(Figure 7.11)**.

HUMAN IMMUNODEFICIENCY VIRUS

Human immunodeficiency virus (HIV) is a spherical enveloped virus having single stranded RNA genome.

Reverse transcriptase is associated with viral enzyme and converts RNA into single stranded DNA, which gets integrated into the host cell chromosome. This DNA remains in the latent state for years in the host cells and is the reason for latent infection. HIV is causative agent of acquired immunodeficiency syndrome (AIDS). The virus belongs to retrovirus family and attacks the immune system, which is so important for protection against illness **(Figure 7.12)**.

EBOLA VIRUS

The Ebola virus causes an acute, serious illness which is often fatal if untreated. Ebola virus disease (EVD) first appeared in 1976 in 2 simultaneous outbreaks, one in what is now, Nzara, South Sudan, and the other in Yambuku, Democratic Republic of Congo. The latter occurred in a village near the Ebola River, from which the disease takes its name. The 2014–2016 outbreak in West Africa was the largest and most complex Ebola outbreak since the virus was first discovered in 1976. There were more cases and deaths in this outbreak than all others combined **(Figure 7.13)**.

Ebola is introduced into the human population through close contact with the blood, secretions, organs or other bodily fluids of infected animals such as chimpanzees, gorillas, fruit bats, monkeys, forest antelope and porcupines found ill or dead or in the rainforest.

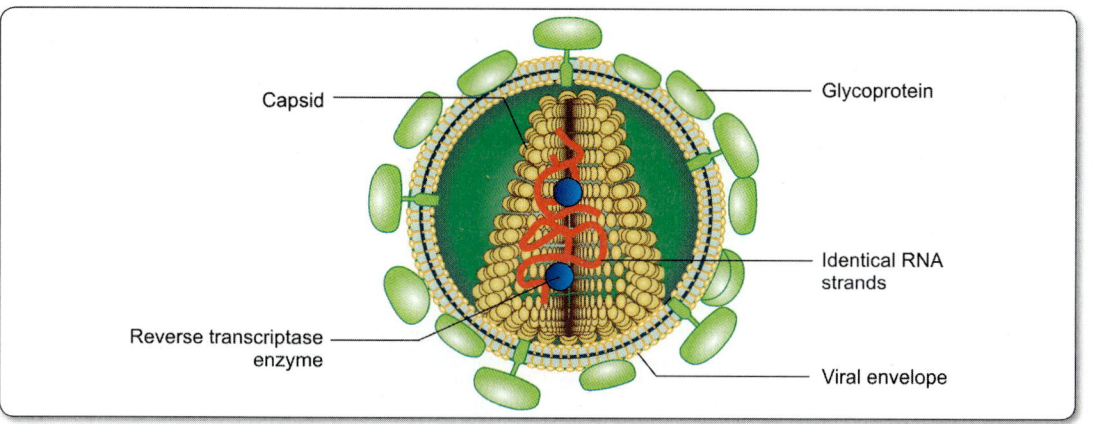

Figure 7.12: Human immunodeficiency virus

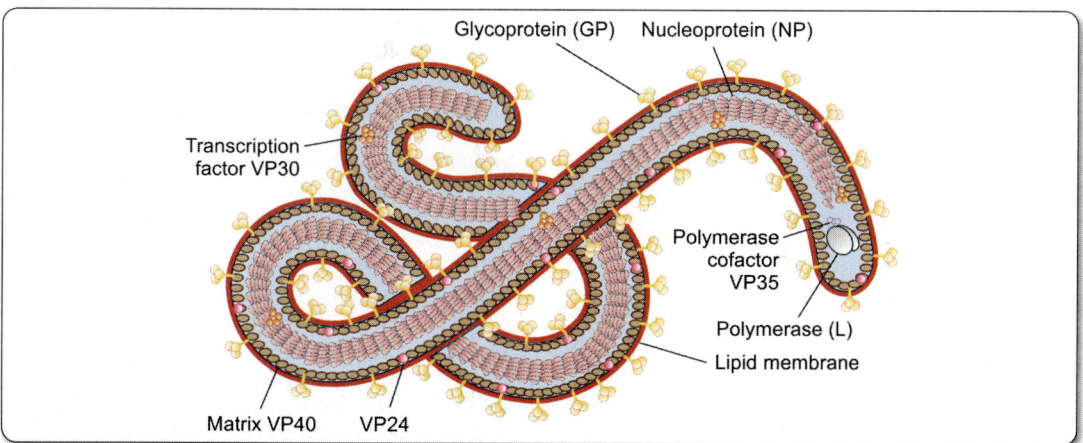

Figure 7.13: Ebola virus

DENGUE VIRUS

The dengue viruses are members of the genus Flavivirus in the family Flaviviridae. The dengue virus genome is a single strand of RNA.

Dengue infections are caused by four closely related viruses named DEN-1, DEN-2, DEN-3, and DEN-4. These four viruses are called serotypes because each has different interactions with the antibodies in human blood serum. The four dengue viruses are similar—they share approximately 65% of their genomes—but even within a single serotype, there is some genetic variation. Despite these variations, infection with each of the dengue serotypes results in the same disease and range of clinical symptoms. The fever caused by dengue virus is painful and is also known as break bone fever (**Figure 7.14**).

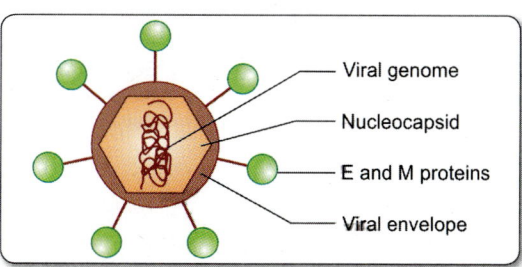

Figure 7.14: Dengue virus

ZIKA VIRUS

The disease is transmitted by infected *Aedes aegypti* mosquito. The infection can be passed on to the fetus *in utero* and could lead to serious birth defects. The infection can also be transmitted sexually if one of the partners is having Zika infection, it may be symptomatic or asymptomatic at the time of transmission of infection. The symptoms are like that of mild form of dengue. There are no medicines and vaccines for this disease and it can be prevented by avoiding mosquito bite and refraining from visiting areas having this disease.

COMMON VIRAL DISEASES

Common viral diseases are summarized in **Table 7.1**.

TABLE 7.1: **Common Viral Diseases**

Disease	Caused by	Spread	Symptoms
AIDS	Human immunodeficiency virus (HIV)	Blood exchange	Severely weakens immunity and makes way for a number of other pathogens.
Chicken pox	Varicella zoster virus (VZV)	Air/contact	Chicken pox, also known as varicella, is a highly contagious disease. The disease results in a characteristic skin rash that forms small, itchy blisters. Less severe than small pox. Almost eradicated after the invention of vaccination.
Smallpox	Variola major and Variola minor	Air/contact/water	One of the highly dreaded diseases that is highly contagious. Almost eradicated after the invention of vaccination.
Chikungunya	Chikungunya virus	*Aedes* mosquitoes, such as *A. aegypti* and *A. albopictus*	Causes severe joint pains. Animal reservoirs of the virus include monkeys, birds, cattle, and rodents. This is in contrast to dengue, for which primates are the only hosts
Cold, influenza (flu) and most coughs	Rhino viruses	Air borne droplets of sneeze	Summer are hostile for the virus. Most common during winter months.
Dengue fever	Flavivirus	Female Aedes mosquito	High fever, headache, vomiting, muscle and joint pains, and a characteristic skin rash. In a small proportion of cases, the disease develops into the life-threatening dengue hemorrhagic fever, resulting in bleeding, **low levels of blood platelets** and blood plasma leakage, or into dengue shock syndrome, where dangerously low blood pressure occurs.
Ebola	Ebola virus	Animal to man	Ebola infection shows a sudden onset of the disease resulting initially in flu-like symptoms: fever, chills and malaise. As the disease progresses, it results in multi-system involvements indicated by the person experiencing lethargy, nausea, vomiting, diarrhea and headache.
Hepatitis B	Hepatitis B virus (HBV)	Blood Exchange, Sexually transmitted disease (STD)	Affects the liver. Acute as well as chronic.
Measles	Measles virus	Air	Complications occur in about 30% and may include diarrhea, blindness, inflammation of the brain, and pneumonia among others
Polio or Polio myelitis	Poliovirus	Water/fecal-oral	Weak muscles leading to deformations
Zika	Zika virus	*Aedes* mosquitoes, such as *A. aegypti* and *A. albopictus*	

Color Plates of Viral Diseases

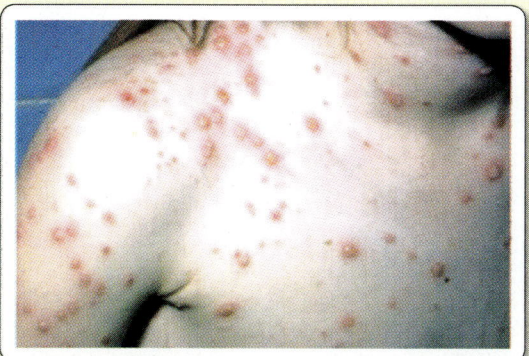

Color plate 1: Chicken pox

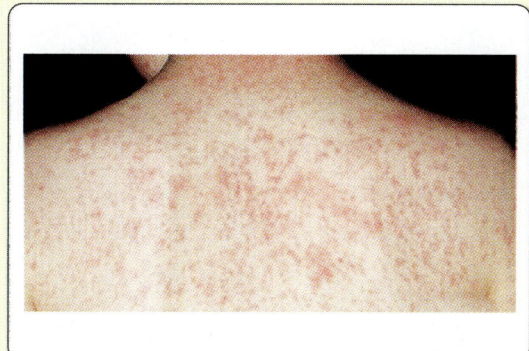

Color plate 2: Measles

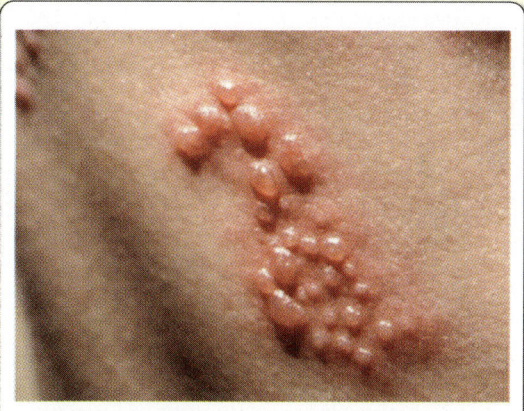

Color plate 3: Shingles

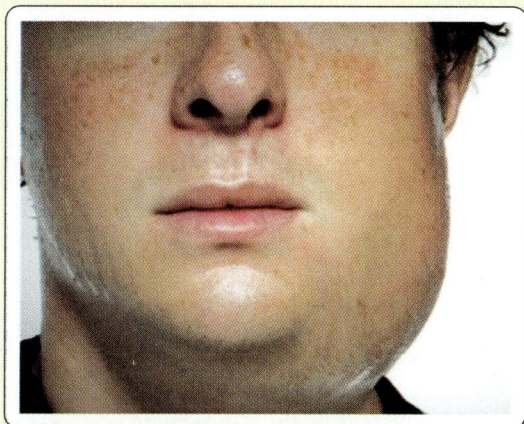

Color plate 4: Mumps

Assess Yourself

LONG ANSWER QUESTIONS

1. Write about pathogenicity of AIDS
2. Discuss rabies

MULTIPLE CHOICE QUESTIONS

1. HIV is a:
   a. Retrovirus
   b. DNA virus
   c. Fungus
   d. Bacteria

2. Most effective mode of transmission of HIV:
   a. Sexual
   b. Blood product
   c. Needle/syringe
   d. Mother of fetus

3. Hepatitis virus that spreads by fecal-oral route:
   a. Hepatitis A
   b. Hepatitis B
   c. Hepatitis C
   d. Hepatitis D

4. The causative agent of AIDS is:
   a. Human immunodeficiency virus (HIV)
   b. *Mycobacterium tuberculosis*
   c. *Mycobacterium leprae*
   d. *Treponema pallidum*

5. Dengue is caused by:
   a. Alphavirus
   b. Bunyavirus
   c. Flavivirus
   d. Hantavirus

6. Rabies is a ------ disease.
   a. Zoonotic
   b. Parasitic
   c. Bacterial
   d. None of the above

ANSWERS TO MCQs

1. a   **2.** b   **3.** a   **4.** a   **5.** c   **6.** a

Common Fungal Diseases

INTRODUCTION

Fungi play key roles in many biological processes, including many processes that support, and in other cases adversely affect other forms of life. The word *fungus* comes from the Latin word that means mushroom.

The kingdom Fungi includes an enormous variety of living organisms collectively referred to as Ascomycota, or true Fungi. While scientists have identified about 100,000 species of fungi, this is only a fraction of the 1.5 million species of fungus probably present on earth. Edible mushrooms, yeasts, black mold, and the producer of the antibiotic penicillin, *Penicillium notatum*, are all members of the kingdom Fungi.

IMPORTANT CHARACTERISTICS

Fungi are cosmopolitan, i.e. they are found all over the world and occur in air, water, soil and on plants and animals. They prefer to grow in warm and humid places. They do not contain chlorophyll, hence, are non-photosynthetic. Most of the fungi are multicellular (hyphae); however, some are unicellular (yeast). They are non-motile and their cell walls made of chitin instead of cellulose like that of a plant.

They are absorptive heterotrophs i.e. they digest food externally and then absorb it.

STRUCTURE OF FUNGI

Being eukaryotes, a typical fungal cell contains a true nucleus and many membrane-bound organelles. The body of the fungus is made of tiny filaments or tubes called hyphae. They contain cytoplasm and nuclei (>1). Each hyphae is one continuous cell and their cell wall made of chitin **(Figure 8.1)**. A tangled mess of hyphae is called mycelium. Rhizoids are root-like parts of fungi that anchor them to the substrate (whatever they are bonding to). Mycelium increase the surface area of the fungi to absorb more nutrients.

REPRODUCTION

A single fungus may reproduce by both asexual and sexual mode. Reproduction involves formation of asexual and sexual spores.

- **Sexual reproduction** involves a union between two nuclei or two sex cells or two sex organs. A zygote is formed and meiotic divisions take place that result in formation of spores. These spores are capable of giving rise to new fungal organism when suitable conditions are found.

Section II • Microorganisms

- **Asexual reproduction** is the main method of reproduction and it includes:
  - Fragmentation of hyphae and each fragment grows into a new individual fungus.
  - Fission of a mature cell into two by binary fission.
  - Budding of cells in which each bud produces new individual.

MORPHOLOGICAL CLASSIFICATION

On the basis of morphology, there are four groups of fungi:

- **Yeasts:** Yeasts are round, oval or elongated unicellular fungi. Most of them reproduce by an asexual process called budding in which the cell develops a protuberance, which enlarges and eventually separates from the parent cell **(Figures 8.1A and B).**
- **Yeast-like:** In some yeasts like *Candida*, the bud remains attached to the mother cell and elongates, followed by repeated budding forming chains of elongated cells known as pseudohyphae. These can be differentiated from true hyphae because they have constriction at the septa and the septa are also present at the branching point **(Figure 8.1C).** Some species like *C. albicans* also produce true hyphae.
- **Molds:** In molds, spores germinate to produce branching filaments called hyphae (singular hypha). They are 2–10 µm in diameter **(Figures 8.1D and E).** They may be septate or nonseptate (coenocytic). The hyphae continue

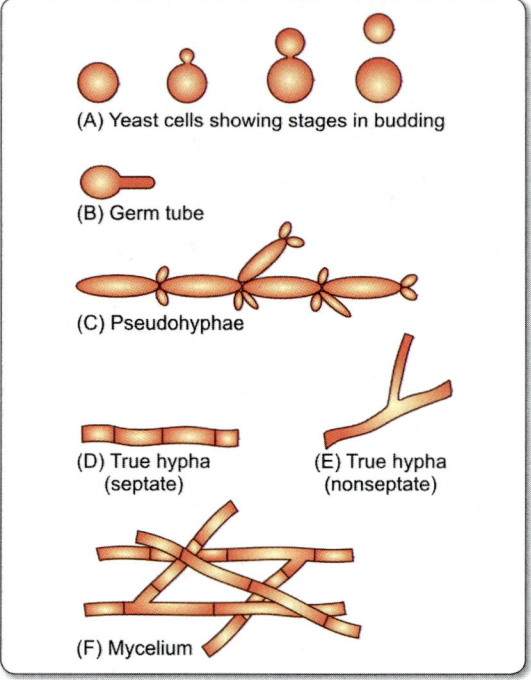

(A) Yeast cells showing stages in budding

(B) Germ tube

(C) Pseudohyphae

(D) True hypha (septate)   (E) True hypha (nonseptate)

(F) Mycelium

Figures 8.1A to F: Basic fungal morphology

to grow **(Figure 8.1F)** and branch to form tangled mass of growth called mycelium.

- **Dimorphic fungi:** Many fungi pathogenic to man have a yeast form in the host tissue and in vitro at 37°C on enriched media, and hyphal (mycelial) form *in vitro* at 25°C. These are known as dimorphic fungi.

COMMON FUNGAL DISEASES

Common fungal diseases are summarized in Table 8.1.

TABLE 8.1: Invasive Fungal Infections, Pathogens and Characteristics of Disease

Disease type	Causative agent	Clinical signs and symptoms
Candidiasis	*Candida* species	• Acute disseminated: fever, chills, polymyalgia, polyarthralgia, not tender pinkish skin lesions, retinal exudates • Chronic: complaints of the organ involved
Aspergillosis	*Aspergillus* species	• Unremitting fever and pulmonary infiltrates during antibiotic therapy. Chest pain, pleural rub, pleural effusion, hemoptysis. Halo and air crescent sign on chest radiograph and CT scan • Clinical and radiologic sinusitis

Contd…

Disease type	Causative agent	Clinical signs and symptoms
Cryptococcosis	*Cryptococcus neoformans*	• Flu-like symptoms; skin lesions, headache without meningismus
Zygomycosis	*Rhizopus* species *Absidia* species *Mucor* species	• Like aspergillosis, more outspoken rhinocerebral form with serosanguinous nasal discharge
Others	*Malassezia furfur*	• Often catheter-associated; pneumonia
	Trichosporon species	• Skin and lung lesions
	Fusarium species	
	Pseudallescheria boydii	• Often positive blood cultures. • Skin lesions, severe myalgia. • Abscess formation with symptoms depending on organ involved
	Scedosporium species	• Like aspergillosis; wound infections
	Alternaria species	
Blastomyscosis	*Blastomyces dermatitidis*	• Ulcerative lesions; skin, urogenital tract • Central nervous system
Histoplasmosis	*Histoplasma capsulatum*	• Pulmonary infiltrates; mucocutaneous ulcers • Hepatosplenomegaly
Coccidiomycosis	*Coccidioidis immitis*	• Pulmonary infection. • Dissemination with osteomyelitis, arthritis, meningitis
Para-coccidiomycosis	*Paracoccidioidis brasiliensis*	• Pulmonary infection. • Dissemination to skin, mucosa and lymphnodes
Penicilliosis	*Penicillium marneffei*	• Skin and subcutaneous lesions, lymphadenitis, splenomegaly

RING WORM INFECTION

- A highly contagious fungal infection of the skin or scalp.
- Ringworm is caused by a type of fungus that eats keratin. These are called dermatophytes.
- Dermatophytes attack the skin, scalp, hair, and nails because those are the only parts of the body with enough keratin to attract them.
- Ringworm is spread by skin-to-skin contact or by touching an infected animal or object.
- Ringworm is typically scaly and may be red and itchy. Ringworm of the scalp is common in children, where it may cause bald patches.
- The treatment for ringworm is antifungal medication like terbinafine.

ATHLETE'S FOOT

- A fungal infection that usually begins between the toes.
- Athlete's foot commonly occurs in people whose feet have become very sweaty while confined within tight-fitting shoes.
- Symptoms include a scaly rash that usually causes itching, stinging and burning. People with athlete's foot can have moist, raw skin between their toes.
- If untreated, athlete's foot can result in a bacterial infection if skin is broken. This can happen due to scratching or when blisters pop or ulcers become infected. It is very serious and requires prompt treatment. Athlete's foot is also very contagious.

Color Plates of Common Fungal Diseases

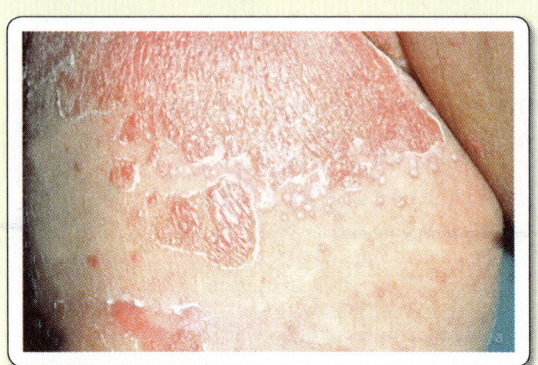

Color plate 1: Candidiasis

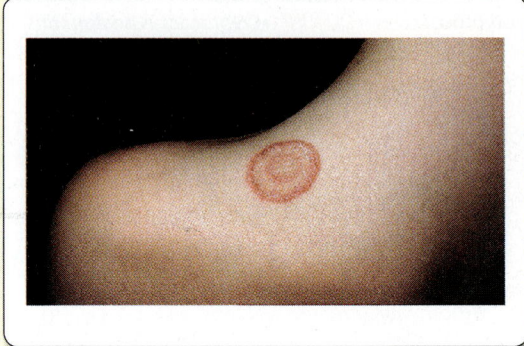

Color plate 2: Ring worm infection

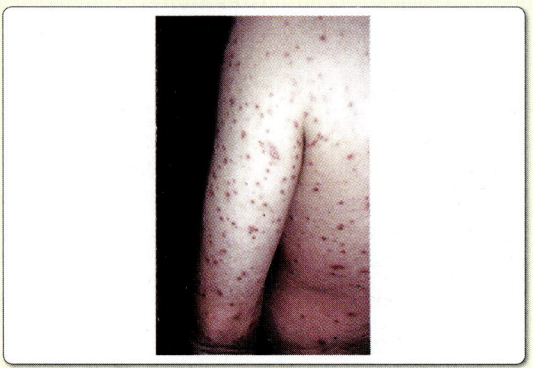

Color plate 3: Histoplasmosis

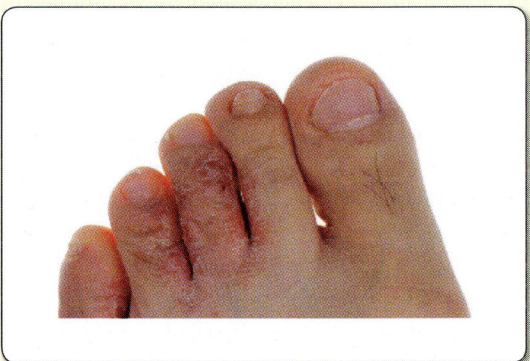

Color plate 4: Athletes foot

Assess Yourself

SHORT NOTES

1. Ring worm infection
2. Aspergillosis
3. Candidiasis

MULTIPLE CHOICE QUESTIONS

1. A tangled mass of hyphae is called:
   - a. Rhizoid
   - b. Mycelium
   - c. Black mold
   - d. None of the above

2. Dimorphic fungi have hyphal form at what temperature?
   - a. 37°C
   - b. 42°C
   - c. 25°C
   - d. 50°C

3. Zygomycosis is caused by all except:
   - a. *Apsergillus*
   - b. *Rhizopus*
   - c. *Mucor*
   - d. *Absidia*

4. Candidiasis is caused by:
   - a. Candida albicans
   - b. Rhizopus
   - c. Aspergillus
   - d. None of the above

5. Fungal infections are most commonly seen in people having:
   - a. Weak immune system
   - b. Unhygienic habits
   - c. Organ transplant
   - d. All of the above

6. The fungal infections are most common in people who live in:
   - a. Warm places
   - b. Moist places
   - c. On creased areas of body
   - d. All of the above

ANSWERS TO MCQS

1. b   **2.** c   **3.** a   **4.** a   **5.** d   **6.** d

Chapter

9

Common Parasitic Diseases

INTRODUCTION

A parasite is an organism that lives on or in a host organism and gets its food from or at the expense of its host. There are three main classes of parasites that can cause disease in humans: protozoa, helminths, and ectoparasites.

Terms to Learn

- **Ectoparasite:** Parasites that live outside the body
- **Endoparasite:** Parasites that live inside the body
- **Parasitism:** It is a situation where parasite is benefitted from the host and completely lives on the nourishment obtained from the body of the host.
- **Host:** This is a body in which a parasite lives in order to derive nourishment and shelter. The host suffers due to harmful activities of the parasite.
- **Definitive host:** The host in which the parasites spend the adult phase of their life cycle in the body of human or they may utilize human body to complete sexual stage of their life cycle.
- **Intermediate host:** The host in which a parasite completes asexual phase of its life cycle.

PROTOZOANS

Protozoa are microscopic, one-celled organisms that can be free-living or parasitic in nature. They are able to multiply in humans, which contributes to their survival and also permits serious infections to develop from just a single organism. Transmission of protozoa that live in a human's intestine to another human typically occurs through a fecal-oral route (for example, contaminated food or water or person-to-person contact). Protozoa that live in the blood or tissue of humans are transmitted to other humans by an arthropod vector (for example, through the bite of a mosquito or sand fly).

Entamoeba histolytica

Entamoeba histolytica is a protozoan parasite responsible for a disease called amoebiasis. It occurs usually in the large intestine and causes internal inflammation as its name suggests. Inside humans, *Entamoeba histolytica* lives and multiplies as a trophozoite. Trophozoites are oblong and about 15–20 μm in length. In order to infect other humans, they encyst and exit the body (**Figures 9.1A to E**).

Pseudopodium
Endoplasm
Ingested erythrocytes
Ectoplasm
Nucleus
A
B
Chromidial bar
Glycogen mass
C
D
E

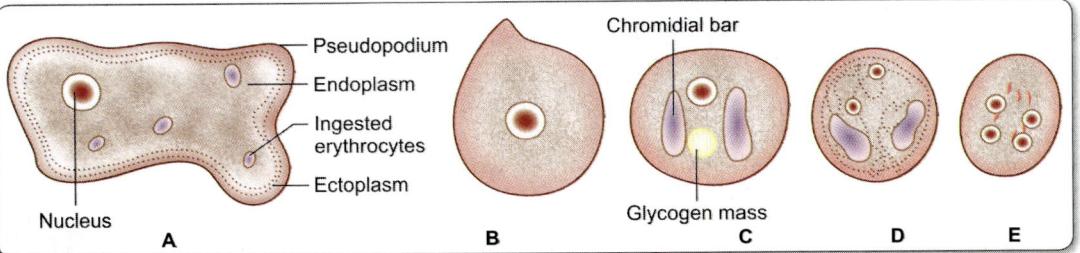

Figures 9.1A to E: Various morphological forms of *Entamoeba histolytica*. A. Trophozoite, B. Precystic stage, C. Uninucleate cyst, D. Binucleate cyst, E. Mature quadrinucleate cyst

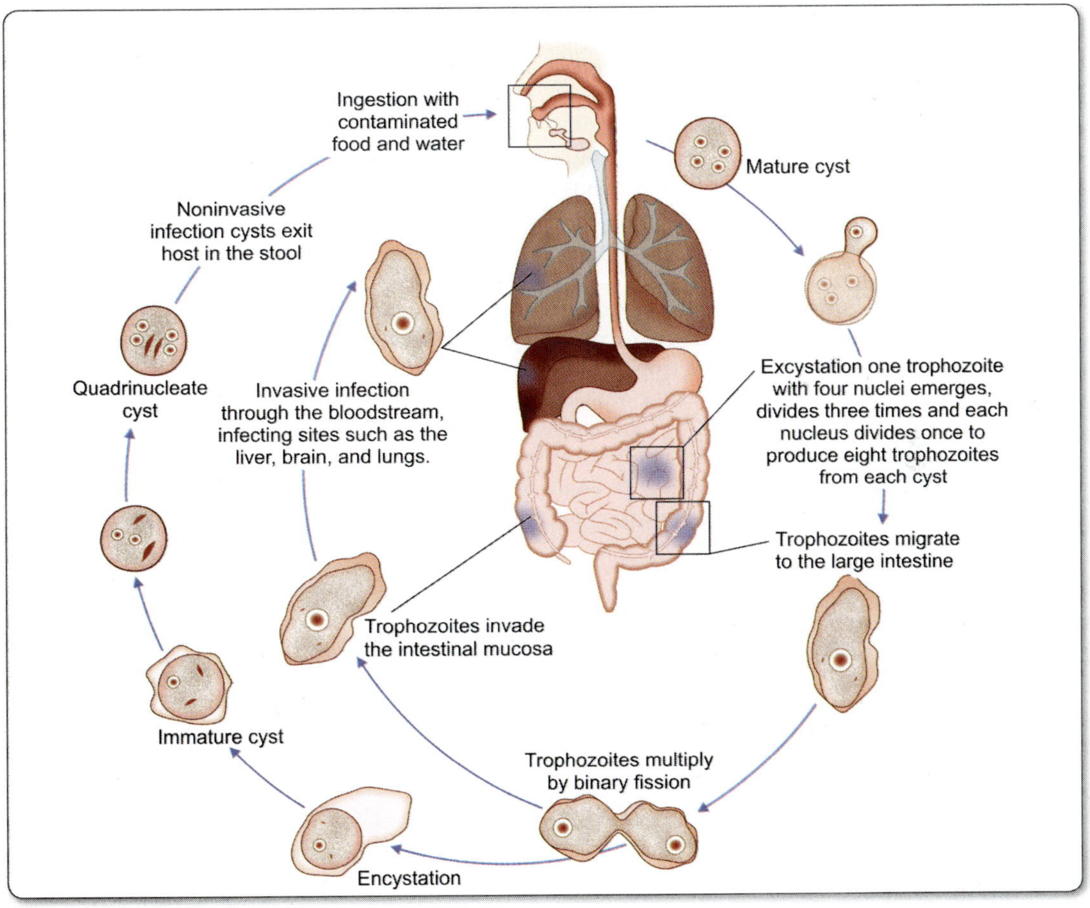

Ingestion with contaminated food and water
Mature cyst
Noninvasive infection cysts exit host in the stool
Quadrinucleate cyst
Invasive infection through the bloodstream, infecting sites such as the liver, brain, and lungs.
Excystation one trophozoite with four nuclei emerges, divides three times and each nucleus divides once to produce eight trophozoites from each cyst
Trophozoites migrate to the large intestine
Trophozoites invade the intestinal mucosa
Immature cyst
Trophozoites multiply by binary fission
Encystation

Figure 9.2: Life cycle of *Entamoeba histolytica*

The **life cycle** (Figure 9.2) of *Entamoeba histolytica* does not require any intermediate host. Mature cysts (spherical, 12–15 µm in diameter) are passed in the feces of an infected human. Another

human can get infected by ingesting them in fecally contaminated water, food or hands. If the cysts survive the acidic stomach, they transform back into trophozoites in the small intestine. Trophozoites migrate to the large intestine where they live and multiply by binary fission. Both cysts and trophozoites are sometimes present in the feces.

Giardia lamblia

Giardia is a microscopic parasite that causes the diarrheal illness known as giardiasis. *Giardia* (also known as *Giardia intestinalis*, *Giardia lamblia*, or *Giardia duodenalis*) is found on surfaces or in soil, food, or water that has been contaminated with feces from infected humans or animals.

Giardia is protected by an outer shell that allows it to survive outside the body for long periods of time and makes it tolerant to chlorine disinfection. While the parasite can be spread in different ways, but water (drinking water and recreational water) is the most common mode of transmission.

Giardia lamblia exists in two forms, an active form called a trophozoite, and an inactive form called a cyst **(Figures 9.3A to C)**. The active trophozoite attaches to the lining of the small intestine with a "sucker" and is responsible for causing the signs and symptoms of giardiasis. Cysts of *Giardia* are present in the feces of infected persons. Thus, the infection is spread from person to person by contamination of

food with feces, or by direct fecal-oral contamination. Cysts also survive in water, for example in fresh water lakes and streams. As a result, giardiasis is the most common cause of water-borne, parasitic illness.

Plasmodium

Plasmodium is the causative organism of malaria. *Plasmodium*, which infects red blood cells in mammals (including humans), birds, and reptiles, occurs worldwide, especially in tropical and temperate zones. The organism is transmitted by the bite of the female *Anopheles* mosquito.

Five species cause human malaria: *P. vivax* (producing the most widespread form), *P. ovale* (relatively uncommon), *P. falciparum* (producing the most severe symptoms), *P. malariae*, and *P. knowlesi*.

Plasmodium species exhibit three life-cycle stages—gametocytes, sporozoites, and merozoites **(Figure 9.4)**. Gametocytes within a mosquito develop into sporozoites. The sporozoites are transmitted via the saliva of a feeding mosquito to the human bloodstream. From there, they enter liver parenchyma cells, where they divide and form merozoites.

The merozoites are released into the bloodstream and infect red blood cells. Rapid division of the merozoites results in the destruction of the red blood cells, and the newly multiplied merozoites then infect new red blood cells. Some merozoites may develop

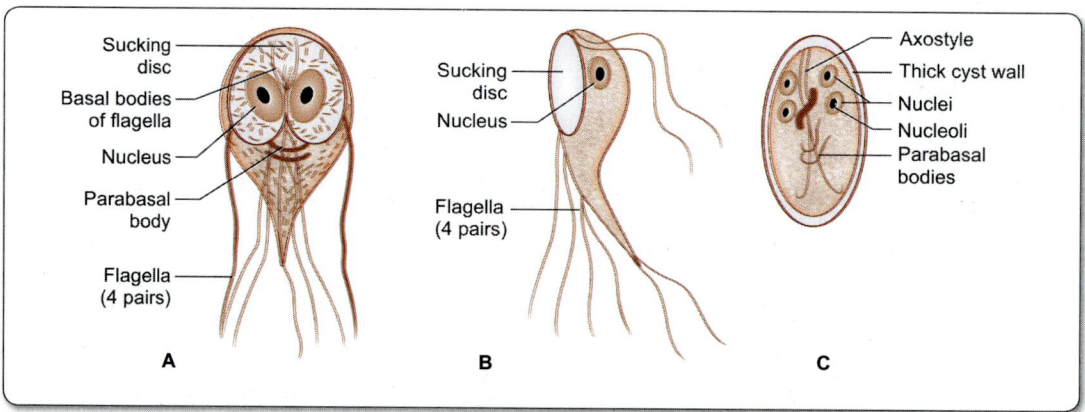

Figures 9.3A to C: Morphological forms of *Giardia lamblia*. A. Trophozoite, B. Lateral view of trophozoite, C. Cyst

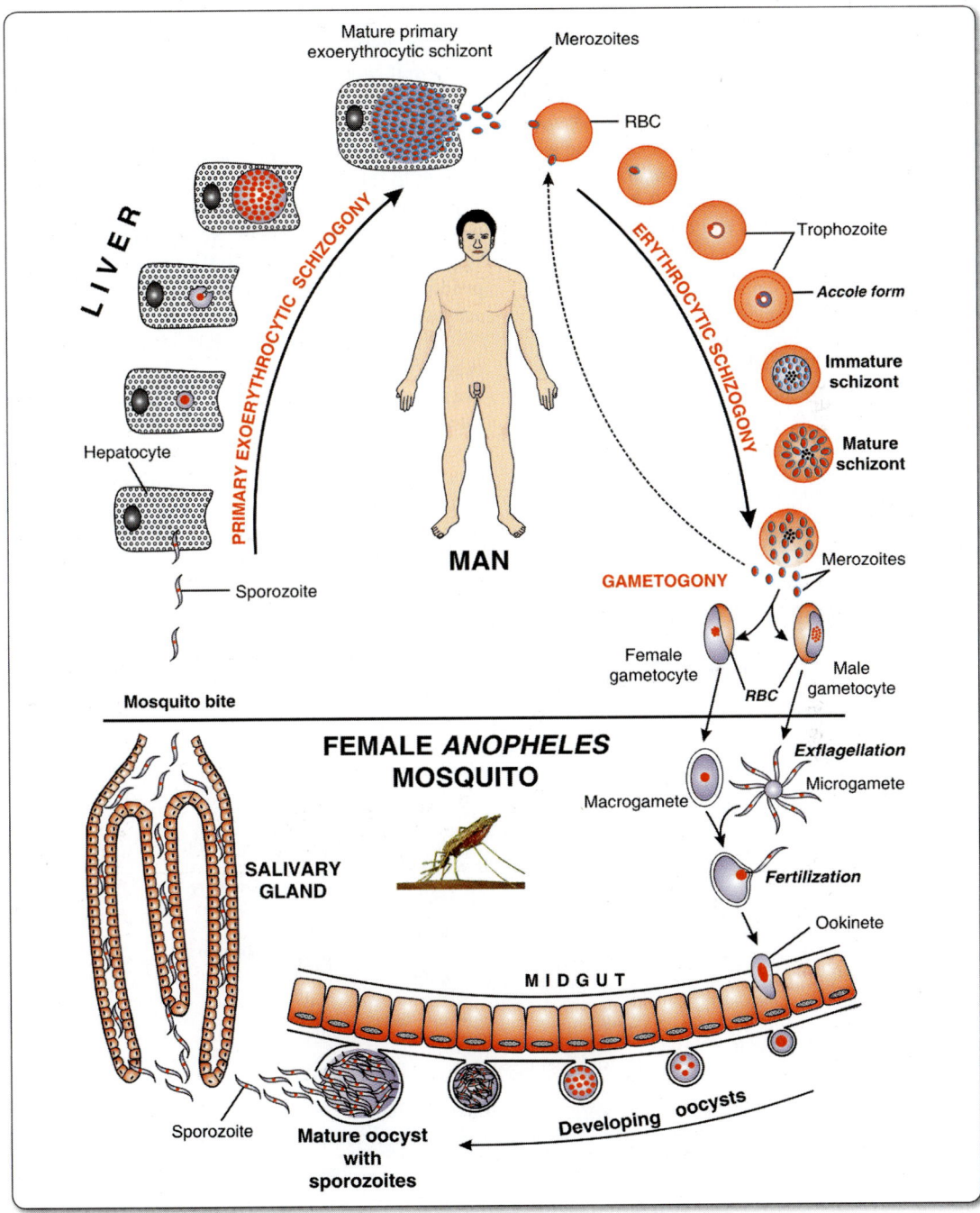

Figure 9.4: Life cycle of malarial parasite

into gametocytes, which can be ingested by a feeding mosquito, starting the life cycle over again. The red blood cells destroyed by the merozoites liberate toxins that cause the periodic chill-and-fever cycles that are the typical symptoms of malaria. *P. vivax*, *P. ovale*, and *P. falciparum* repeat this chill-fever cycle every 48 hours (tertian malaria), and *P. malariae* repeats it every 72 hours (quartan malaria). *P. knowlesi* has a 24-hour life cycle and thus can cause daily spikes in fever.

HELMINTHS

Ascaris lumbricoides

Ascaris lumbricoides, an intestinal roundworm, is one of the most common helminthic human infections worldwide. *A. lumbricoides* is the largest intestinal nematode of man. The female worms are larger than the males and can measure 40 cm in length and 6 mm in diameter. They are white or pink and are tapered at both ends **(Figure 9.5)**.

Transmission occurs mainly via ingestion of water or food (raw vegetables or fruit in particular) contaminated with *A. lumbricoides* eggs and occasionally via inhalation of contaminated dust.

Children playing in contaminated soil may acquire the parasite from their hands.

Adult worms inhabit the lumen of the small intestine, usually in the jejunum or ileum. They have a life span of 10 months to 2 years and then are passed in the stool. When both female and male worms are present in the intestine, each female worm produces approximately 200,000 fertilized ova per day. When infection with only female worms occurs, infertile eggs that do not develop into the infectious stage are produced. With male-only worm infections, no eggs are formed.

The ova are oval, have a thick shell, a mamillated outer coat, and measure 45–70 μm by 35–50 μm. The ova are passed out in the feces, and embryos develop into infective second-stage larvae in the environment in 2–4 weeks (depending upon environmental conditions). When ingested by humans, the ova hatch in the small intestine and release larvae, which penetrate the intestinal wall and migrate hematogenously or via lymphatics to the heart and lungs. Occasionally, larvae migrate to sites other than the lungs, including to the kidney or brain.

Larvae usually reach the lungs by four days after ingestion of eggs. Within the alveoli of the lungs,

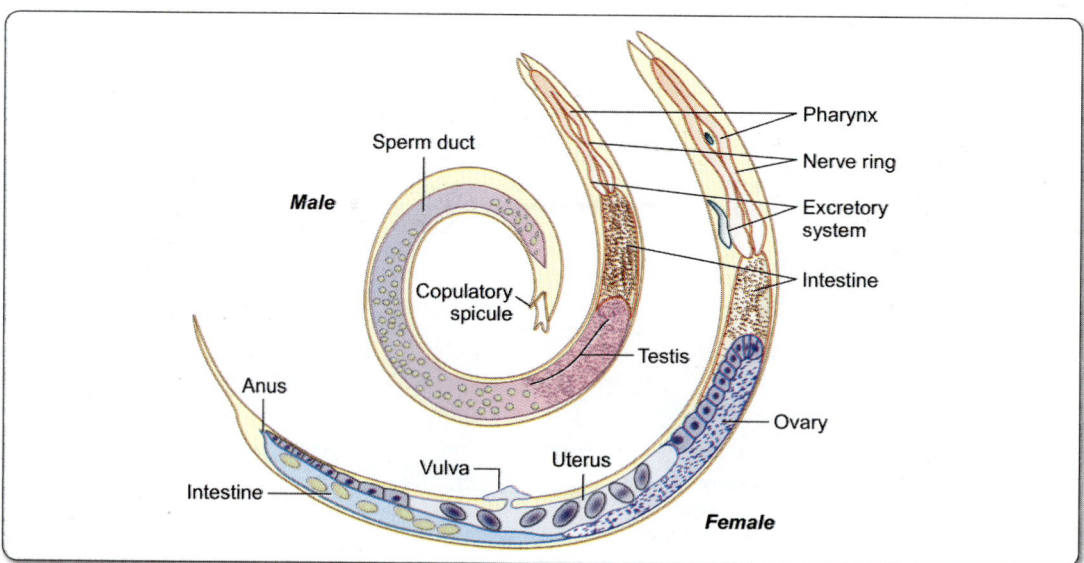

Figure 9.5: Male and female Ascaris

the larvae mature over a period of approximately 10 days, then pass up via bronchi and the trachea, and are subsequently swallowed. Once back in the intestine, they mature into adult worms. Although the majority of worms are found in the jejunum, they may be found anywhere from the esophagus to the rectum. After approximately two to three months, gravid females will begin to produce ova which, when excreted, complete the cycle **(Figure 9.6)**.

Adult worms do not multiply in the human host, so the number of adult worms per infected person relates to the degree of continued exposure to infectious eggs over time.

Ancylostoma duodenale

Ancylostoma duodenale, the Old World hook worm is a very common nematode parasite in the small intestine of man. It causes "ancylostomiasis" in man.

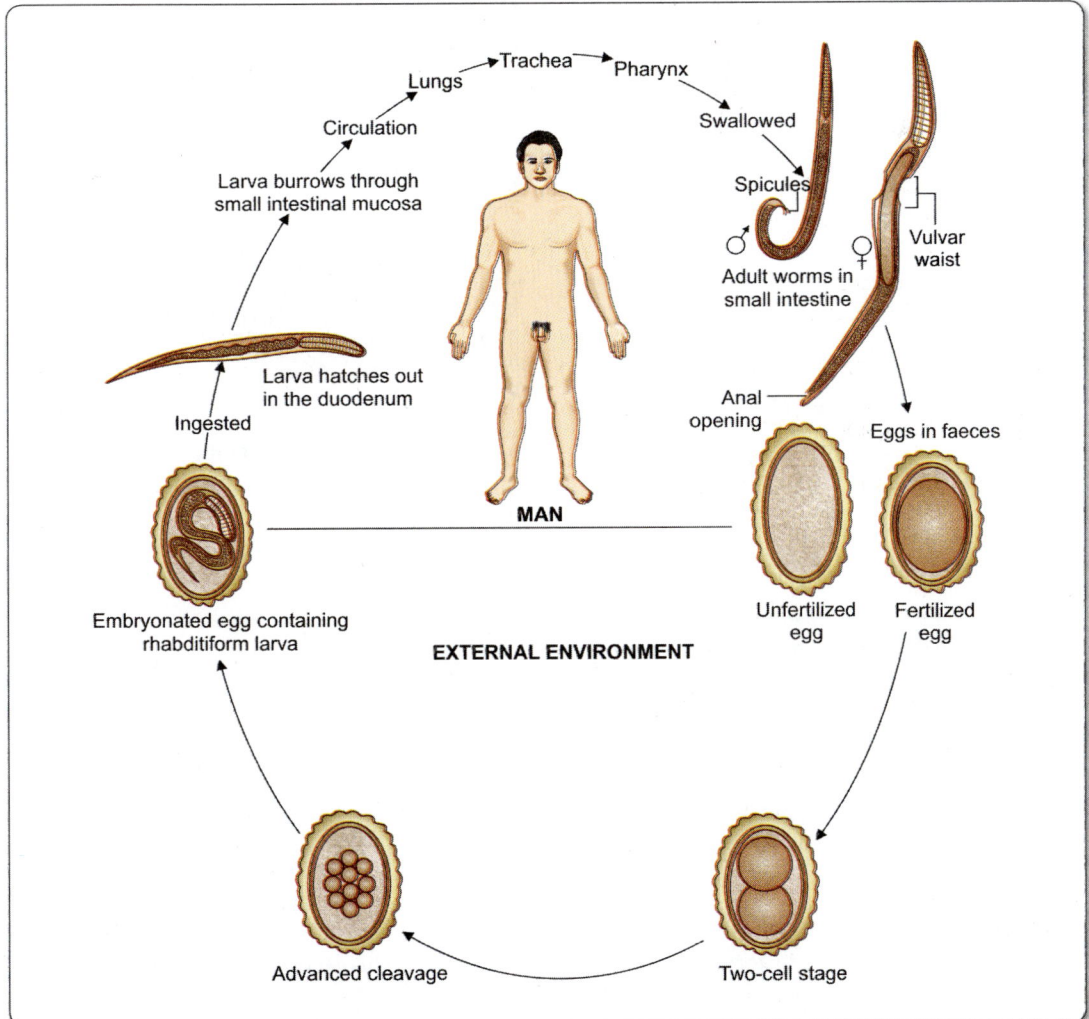

Figure 9.6: Life cycle of *Ascaris lumbricoides*

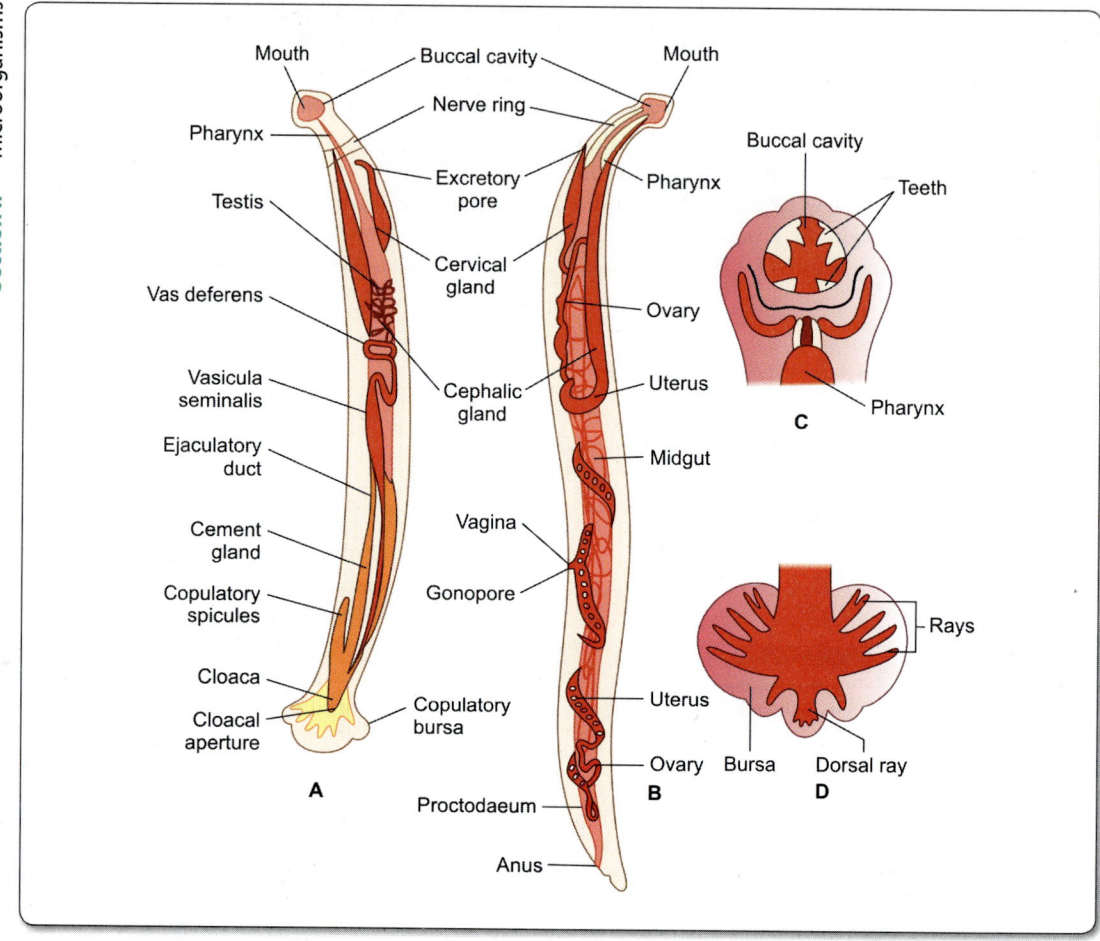

Figures 9.7A to D: *Ancylostoma duodenale.* A. Adult male; B. Adult female; C. Anterior end; D. Posterior end of male

Adult *Ancylostoma duodenale* are small and cylindrical in shape. Sexes are separate; the male is about 8 mm in length and 0.4 mm in diameter, while female is generally longer about 12.5 mm in length and 0.6 mm in diameter. When freshly passed, it has a reddish brown color due to ingested blood in its intestinal tract (**Figures 9.7A to D**).

Copulation occurs in the intestine of the host, during the process the copulatory bursa of male is applied on the vulva of female and sperms are transferred. The female worm lays eggs in the intestine of the host which pass out with feces. On an average nearly 9,000 eggs are laid per day by a female. The eggs, which passed out with the feces, are not infective to man.

Under favorable conditions of environment like moisture, oxygen and temperature, the embryo develops into a rhabditiform larva in the soil. It then develops into a filariform larva measuring about 500–600 pm in length. It is the infective stage of the parasite. This larva does not feed but remains infective and alive for several weeks under favorable conditions. The time taken for development from eggs to filiform larvae, is on an average 8–10 days.

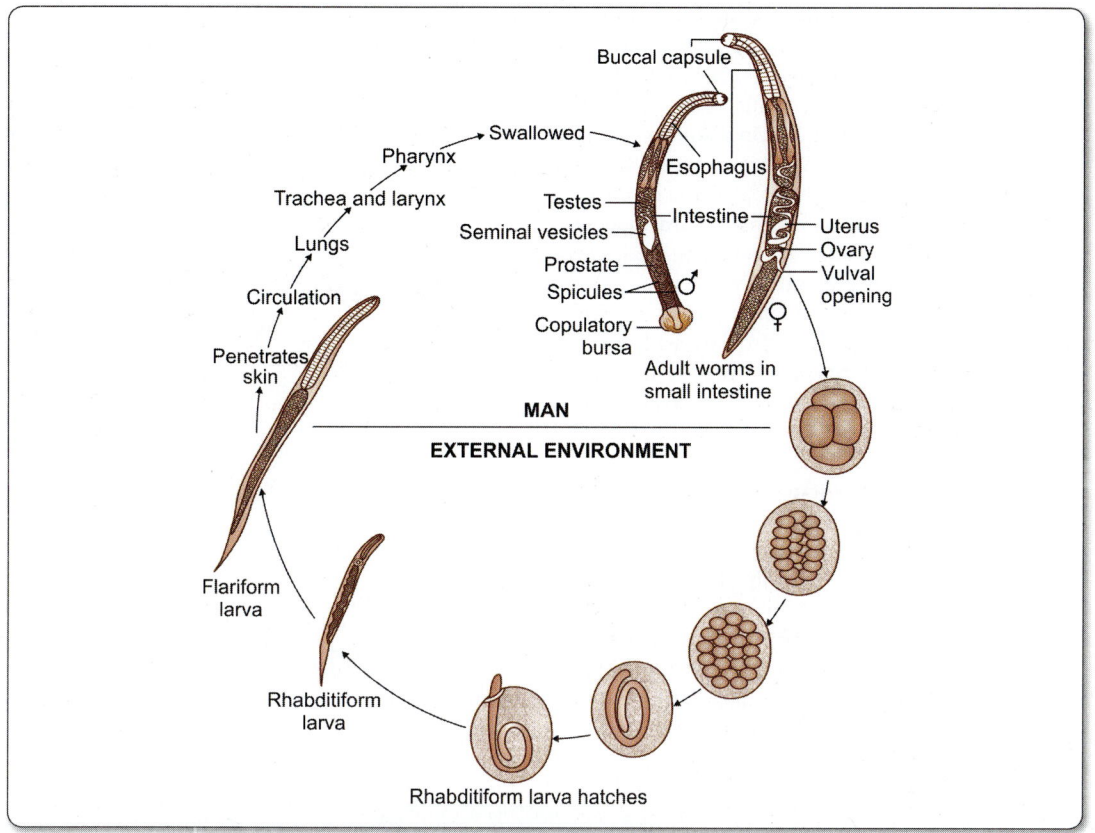

Figure 9.8: Life cycle of *Ancyclostoma duodenale*

The filiform larvae are infective to man. The larvae cast off their sheaths and penetrate the skin of a human host. On reaching the subcutaneous tissues, the larvae enter into the lymphatics and small venules. They pass through the lymphatic-vascular system into the venous circulation and are carried through the right heart into the pulmonary capillaries, where they break through the capillary walls to enter into the alveolar spaces **(Figure 9. 8)**.

They then migrate on the bronchi → trachea → larynx, and crawl over the epiglottis to the back of the pharynx and are finally swallowed. During its migration, when it reaches to esophagus, its third moulting occurs. Thus, finally the growing larvae settle down in the small intestine and undergo fourth and final moult to become the adults.

Wuchereria bancrofti

Wuchereria bancrofti is a parasitic filarial nematode (roundworm) spread by a mosquito vector. It is one of the three parasites that cause lymphatic filariasis, an infection of the lymphatic system by filarial worms. If the infection is left untreated, it can develop into a chronic disease called elephantiasis. *Wuchereria bancrofti* is a dreaded human endoparasite of human blood and lymph.

It is a digenetic parasite completing its life cycle in two hosts. Final host is man, harboring the adult worms, while the intermediate host is blood-sucking mosquito. Adult worms live coiled up in the lymph glands and lymph passages of man, where they often obstruct the flow of lymph.

Adult worms are filiform and cylindrical in shape and both body ends terminate bluntly. They are creamy white in color. Female measures 65–100 mm in length and 0–25 mm in diameter, while male measures 40–50 mm in length and 0–1 mm in diameter.

In human body, the female worm gives birth to embryos, called microfilariae. Microfilariae are born in a very immature stage. They are microscopic, surrounded by a delicate cuticular sheath and containing rudiments of various adult structures **(Figure 9.9)**.

Microfilariae discharged into lymph vessels, soon enter blood vessels and circulate with blood showing active movements. They migrate to reside ultimately in deeper blood vessels of thorax, but they do not undergo further development until sucked by the intermediate host, i.e. mosquito.

Filariasis is caused by blockage of lymph channels by *Wuchereria bancrofti*, the young accumulating in blood vessels near the skin. These elongate, thread-like worms live in the lymphatic system, where they block the vessels. Because lymphatic vessels return tissue fluids to the circulatory system, when the filarial worms block these vessels, fluid tend to accumulate in peripheral tissues. This fluid accumulation causes the enlargement of various appendages, a condition called elephantiasis.

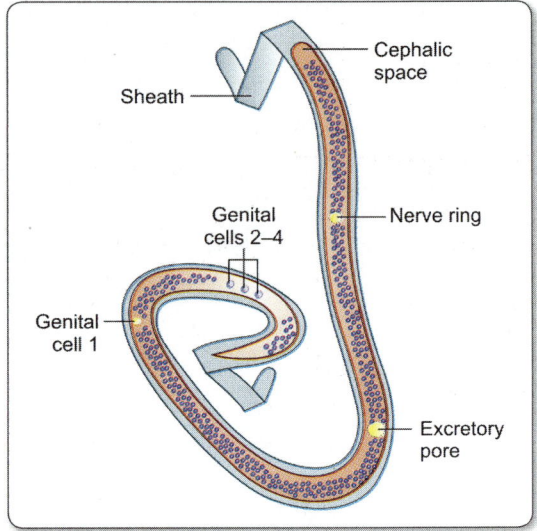

Figure 9.9: *Microfilaria bancrofti*

COMMON DISEASES OF PROTOZOANS AND HELMINTHS

Common diseases caused by protozoans and helminths are summarized in **Tables 9.1 and 9.2**.

TABLE 9.1: Common Diseases caused by Protozoans

Disease	Pathogenic agent	Symptoms	Detection/ identification	Treatment	Source of infection/ prevention
Amebiasis	*Entamoeba histolytica*	Without clinical symptoms or dysentery, flatulence (inflation of the intestine), loss of water, thirst, severe depression, gut ulceration, enlarged liver, hepatic abscesses, death within 4 weeks	Microscopically in sample of feces	*Metronidazole;* 10 mg/kg *Carnidazole* for three days, *Diiodohydroxy-quin,* 20 mg/kg twice per day for three weeks	Usually in feces, water, salad and fruits should be washed
Balantidiasis	*Balantidium coli*	Ulcerative enteritis (inflammation of the intestine), colitis with abundant mucus, but seldom bloody, severe dysentery in humans, usually has little effect on nonhuman primates	Microscopically in sample of feces	*Diiodohydroxy-quin* 20 mg/kg twice per day for three weeks	

Contd...

Disease	Pathogenic agent	Symptoms	Detection/ identification	Treatment	Source of infection/ prevention
Trichomoniasis	*Trichomonas* (for example *Tritichomonas gastritis*)	Pneumonia (*T. tenax, T. hominis*)	Microscopically	*Metronidazole*	Common in birds
Giardiasis	*Giardia*	Bloody diarrhea, sometimes vomiting	In feces	*Metronidazole;* 10 mg/kg	Direct infection; no other host necessary
Cryptosporidiosis	*Cryptosporidium sp.* (*C. parvum*)	Infections most frequent in juveniles and in cases of immunodeficiency; secondary infection due to disease from other pathogenic agents which influence the immune system. Symptoms: gastroenteritis, diarrhea, indigestion, loss of weight, sometimes colic, disturbance of motility. Abdominal seizures.	Detection of *oocysts* in feces; histologically: pathogenic agents visible (dark spots), fixed to the intestinal epithelium or the epithelium of the gall bladder	In humans: no chemotherapy known; typical medicines against Coccidiosis and amoeba are ineffective	Common; mainly oral infection from feces of infected calves. Sick animals emit larger quantities of *oocysts*, especially in the middle of the 14-day-period of disease; in sufficient humidity these remain infectious for 6 months.

TABLE 9.2: Common Diseases caused by Helminths

Disease	Causative agent(s)	Mode of transmission	Laboratory tests	Symptoms	Treatments
Ascariasis	*Ascaris lumbricoides*	Eggs in fecally contaminated food or water	Microscopic examination of the stool, imaging	Shortness of breath, cough, nausea, diarrhea, blood in stool, abdominal pain, weight loss, fatigue	Self-limiting within 1–2 years; albendazole and mebendazole if needed
Hookworm	*Necator americanus, Ancyclostoma duodenale*	Larvae in soil contaminated by dog or cat feces penetrate skin	Microscopic examination of stool (may require a concentration procedure)	Cough, itchy rash, loss of appetite, abdominal pain, diarrhea; in children, may affect physical and congnitive growth	Albendazole and mebendazole; pyrantel pamoate may if needed

Contd...

Disease	Causative agent(s)	Mode of transmission	Laboratory tests	Symptoms	Treatments
Strongyloidiasis	*Strongyloides stercoralis*	Soil-dwelling larvae penetrate the skin, usually bare feet	Microscopic examination of stool over several days (ideally at least 7); some serologic testing available	Often asymptomatic; cough (sometimes bloody), skin rash, abdominal pain, and diarrhea; in immunosuppressed patient, may become disseminated, causing serious and potentially fatal complications	Ivermectin (preferred), albendazole
Enterobiasis (pinworm)	*Enterobius vermicularis*	Fecal-oral route	Observation of eggs or worms from anal area; examination of samples under fingernails	Itching around the anus, abdominal pain, insomnia, irritation of female genital tract	Mebendazole, albendazole, pyrantel pamoate
Trichiuriasis (whipworm)	*Trichuris trichiura*	Fecal contamination of fertilization in soil	Microscopic examination of stool	Abdominal pain, anemia, diarrhea that may be bloody	Albendazole, mebendazole, ivermectin if needed
Trichinosis	*Trichinella spiralis*	Eating raw or undercooked pork or other meat of infected animal	Clinical history, muscle biopsy, serological testing, enzyme immunoassay	Diarrhea, constipation, abdominal pain, headache, cough, chills, light sensitivity, muscle pain, fever, conjunctivitis; in severe cases may affect motor coordination, breathing, heart function	Albendazole, mebendazole if needed
Taeniasis and cysticercosis	*Taenia solium T. saginata T. asiatica Diphyllobothrium latum*	Eating raw or undercooked beef or pork from infected animal	Observation of worm segments or microscopic eggs in stool samples	Asymptomatic or mild GI distress; cysts in muscle, eye, or brain (cysticercosis); brain cysts can cause headaches, seizures, or death	Praziquantel or niclosamide

Contd...

Section II • Microorganisms

Disease	Causative agent(s)	Mode of transmission	Laboratory tests	Symptoms	Treatments
Cystic echinococcosis (hydatid disease)	*Echinococcus granulosus* (cystic)	Exposure to eggs in feces of infected dogs or livestock	Imaging; serological testing including ELISA and indirect hemagglutinin test	Cysts in lungs, liver, and other organs causing nausea, GI distress, and weight loss; severe anaphylaxis or death if cysts burst	Surgical removal or aspiration of cysts or chemotherapy with albendazole or mebenazole
Liver fluke infections	*Fasciola hepatica F. gigantica Clonorchis sinensis Opisthorchis viverrini, O. felineus*	Eating raw or undercooked aquatic plants (*Fasciola* spp.) or freshwater fish (*Clonorchis* spp.) contaminated with eggs or cysts	Microscopic examination of eggs in stool or other samples; immunoassays	Fever, malaise, anemia, abdominal symptoms, transaminitis; cholangitis, cirrhosis, pancreatitis, cholecystitis, gall stones in chronic phase	Triclabendazole (preferred) for *Fasciola* spp.; praziquantel and albendazole for *C. senensis* and *Opisthorchis* spp.
Fasciolopiasis (intestinal fluke)	*Fasciola buski*	Eating raw or undercooked aquatic plants containing cysts	Microscopic examination of eggs in stool or other samples; immunoassays	Diarrhea, abdominal pain; in severe cases, vomiting, nausea, intestinal obstruction, anemia, allergic reactions	Praziquantel

 Assess Yourself

SHORT NOTES

1. Amoebiasis
2. Hydatid disease
3. Tape worm infection

MULTIPLE CHOICE QUESTIONS

1. Ectoparasite lives:
   a. Inside the body
   b. Outside the body
   c. Within the tissues of the body
   d. Don't need any host

2. *E. histolytica* lives inside human body in the form of:
   a. Trophozoite
   b. Uninucleate cyst
   c. Binucleate cyst
   d. Quadrinucleate cyst

Contd...

Assess Yourself

3. *Plasmodium* species exhibits all the stages in its life cycle except:
   a. Gametocytes
   b. Trophozoites
   c. Sporozoites
   d. Merozoites

4. The hook worm is:
   a. *Ascaris lumbricoides*
   b. *Enterobius vermicularis*
   c. *Ancylostoma duodenale*
   d. *Trichuris trichiura*

5. Hydatid disease is caused by:
   a. *Diphyllobothrium*
   b. *Echinococcus*
   c. *Enterobius*
   d. *Fasciola*

6. Malaria is caused by:
   a. Giardia
   b. Plasmodium
   c. None of the above
   d. Both and b

ANSWERS TO MCQS

1. b   2. a   3. b   4. c   5. b   6. b

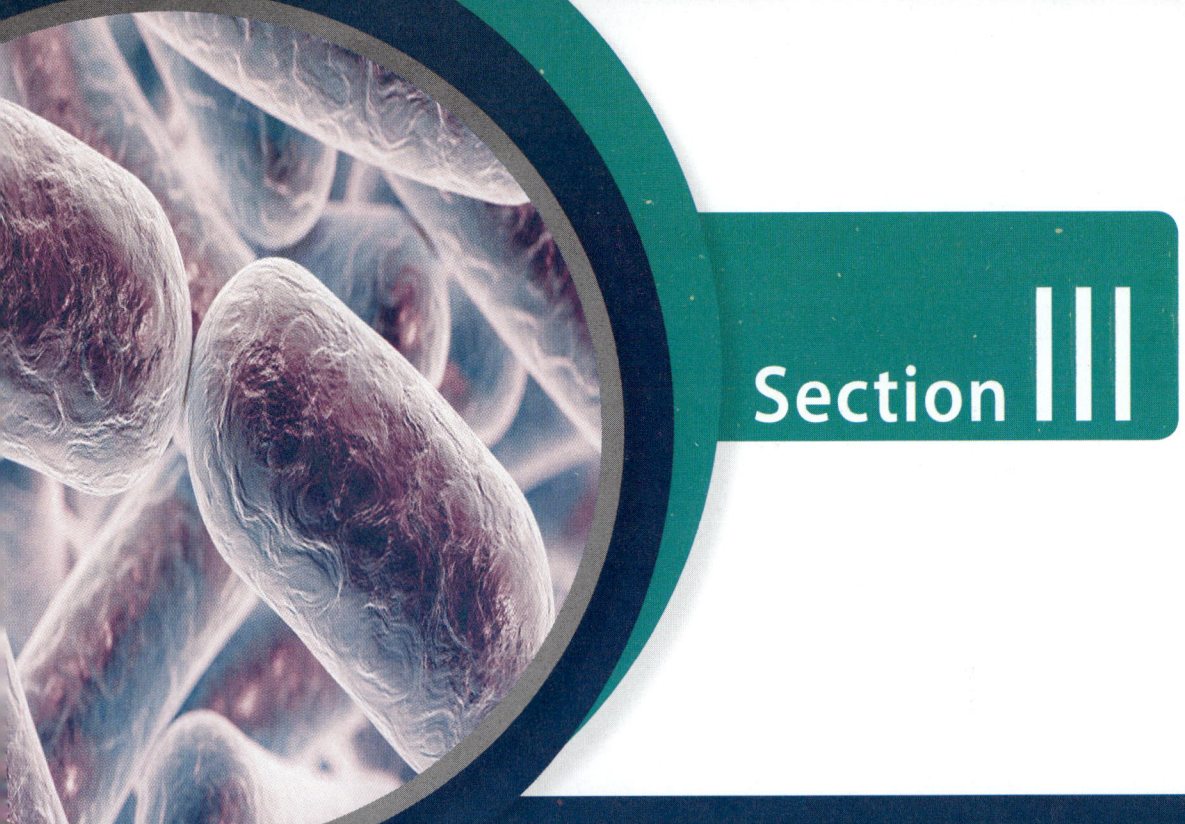

Section III

INFECTIONS AND ITS TRANSMISSION

Section Summary

Infections
(Including Nosocomial Infections)

INTRODUCTION

The invasion and multiplication of microorganisms such as bacteria, viruses, and parasites that are not normally present within the body is known as infection. An infection may cause no symptoms and be subclinical, or it may cause symptoms and be clinically apparent.

Infections can be:
- **Primary infection:** Initial infection caused by a microbe in the host
- **Secondary infection:** Infection caused by another organism in the host when his immunity is lowered down by the primary infection
- **Reinfection:** Infection caused again by the same organism in the same host
- **Nosocomial infection:** Hospital-acquired infection.

SOURCES OF INFECTION

Endogenous Infection

This type of infection may occur in carriers of potentially pathogenic organisms when these previously harmless bacteria invade other surfaces or tissues. A breach in mucosal surfaces often results in infection of the host by members of the normal flora. For example, *Staphylococcus aureus* is a natural inhabitant of nostrils, although it may cause a boil in the skin or infection in a wound.

Exogenous Infection

This type of infection may be acquired in human and animals from outside sources.

Sources of Exogenous Infection

- **Humans:** The most important source of human infection is other humans. Some pathogens like measles are more transmissible than others.
- **Animals:** Animal pathogens may cause infections in humans by direct contact with animals or through the food derived from animals. For example, bovine tuberculosis, anthrax and rabies.
- **Insects:** Insects that feed on blood may transmit a wide range of pathogens. For example, female *Anopheles* mosquitoes transmit malaria to humans while taking blood meal.

- **Soil:** Soil also serves as source of parasitic infection like roundworms and hookworms that are transmitted when the eggs contained in soil (of these parasites) are ingested with eatables.
- **Water:** Water acts as a source of infection when it is contaminated by pathogens like *Vibrio cholerae* due to fecal contamination.
- **Food:** Food may get contaminated by the pathogens or insects like housefly.

PORTALS OF ENTRY

A portal of entry is the site through which microorganisms enter the susceptible host and cause disease/infection. Infectious agents enter the body through various portals, including the mucous membranes, the skin, the respiratory and the gastrointestinal tracts. Pathogens often *enter* the body of the host through the same route they *exited* the reservoir;

for example, airborne pathogens from one person's sneeze can enter through the nose of another person **(Figure 10.1)**.
- Microbes enter the body by various transmission methods
- Most pathogens have specific portals on entry
  - Skin
  - Gastrointestinal tract
  - Respiratory tract
  - Urogenital
  - Placenta.

PORTALS OF EXIT

A portal of exit is the site from where microorganisms leave the host to enter another host and cause disease/infection. For example, a microorganism may leave the reservoir through the nose or mouth when someone sneezes or coughs, or in feces **(Figure 10.2)**.

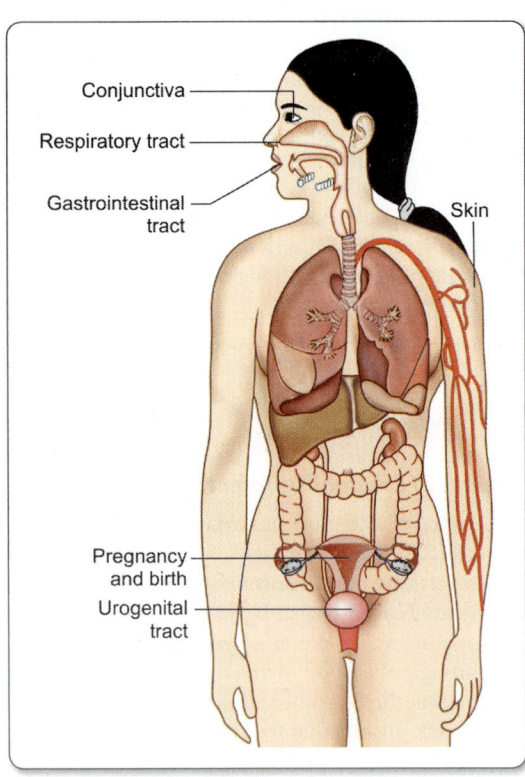

Figure 10.1: Portals of entry

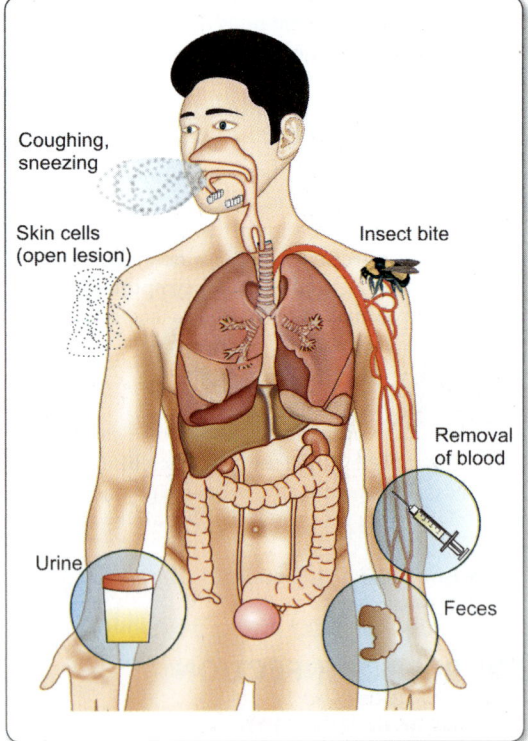

Figure 10.2: Portals of exit

TRANSMISSION OF INFECTION

- Person-to-person spread
  - Direct person-to-person
    - Sexual transmission
    - Perinatal mother to child
    - Needle injection
    - Skin-to-skin
    - Human bites
  - Indirect person-to-person
    - Fomites (contaminated objects)
    - Air: Droplet nuclei (true airborne) and droplets
- Common vehicle spread
  - **Ingested:** Food-borne and water-borne
  - **Biological products:** Vaccines, sera, blood products
- **Zoonoses:** From vertebrate animals
  - Animal bites (e.g., rabies virus or hepatitis from primates)
  - Bloodborne, airborne.
- **Vectorborne:** From insects like mosquitoes, flies, fleas, ticks.

NOSOCOMIAL INFECTIONS

A nosocomial infection—also called "hospital-acquired infection" can be defined as an infection acquired in hospital by a patient, who was admitted for a reason other than that infection or an infection occurring in a patient in a hospital or other healthcare facility in whom the infection was not present or incubating at the time of admission. This includes infections acquired in the hospital but appearing after discharge, and also occupational infections among staff of the facility.

The most common types of nosocomial infections are:

- Urinary tract infections (UTIs)
- Surgical site infections
- Gastroenteritis
- Meningitis
- Pneumonia.

The common bacteria that cause nosocomial infections are listed in **Figure 10.3**.

The nosocomial infections can be identified with various symptoms and findings as listed in **Table 10.1**.

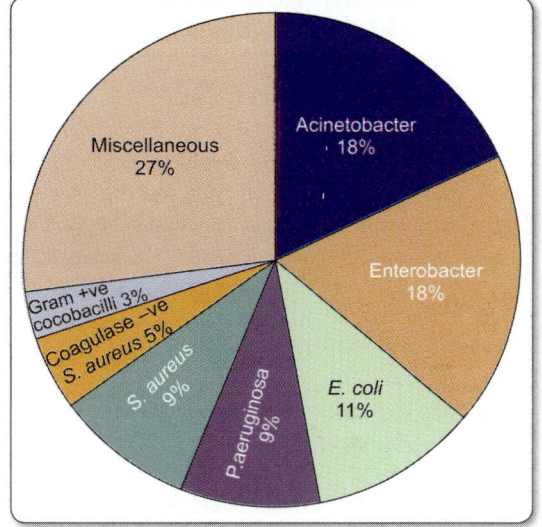

Figure 10.3: Common pathogens causing nosocomial infections

TABLE 10.1: Symptoms and Findings in Nosocomial Infections

Types of nosocomial infection	Symptoms and findings
Surgical site infection	Any purulent discharge, abscess, or spreading cellulitis at the surgical site during the month after the operation
Urinary infection	Positive urine culture (1 or 2 species) with at least 10^5 bacteria/mL, with or without clinical symptoms
Respiratory infection	Respiratory symptoms with at least two of the following signs appearing during hospitalization: —cough— purulent sputum—new infiltrate on chest radiograph consistent with infection

Urinary Infections

This is the most common nosocomial infection; 80% of infections are associated with the use of an indwelling bladder catheter. Urinary infections are associated with less morbidity than other nosocomial infections, but can occasionally lead to bacteremia and death.

Surgical Site Infections

Surgical site infections are also frequent. The incidence varies from 0.5% to 15% depending on the type of operation and underlying patient status. Surgical site infections are a significant problem, which limits the potential benefits of surgical interventions.

Nosocomial Pneumonia

Nosocomial pneumonia occurs in several different patient groups. The most important are patients on ventilators in intensive care units.

Other Nosocomial Infections

These are the four most frequent and important nosocomial infections, but there are many other potential sites of infection. For example:

- **Skin and soft tissue infections:** Open sores (ulcers, burns and bedsores) encourage bacterial colonization and may lead to systemic infection.
- **Gastroenteritis:** It is the most common nosocomial infection in children, where rotavirus is a chief pathogen. *Clostridium difficile* is the major cause of nosocomial gastroenteritis in adults in developed countries.
- Sinusitis and other enteric infections, infections of the eye and conjunctiva.
- Endometritis and other infections of the reproductive organs following childbirth.

REACTION OF BODY TO INFECTION

Infection does not necessarily lead to disease. Microorganisms are capable of causing disease and they usually enter our bodies through the mouth, eyes, nose, or urogenital openings, or through wounds or bites that breach the skin barrier.

In response to infection, immune system comes into action. White blood cells, antibodies, and other mechanisms function to rid your body of the pathogens. In fact many symptoms of an infection such as fever, malaise, headache, and rash are the activities of the immune system that helps to eliminate the infection from the body.

Mechanism of Resistance

The body has defense system that helps it to come over the foreign invaders. The defenses of body are as follows:

- The first line of defense is the physical and chemical barriers, which are functions of innate immunity.
  - **Physical barriers** are physical barriers to invaders.
    - **Skin:** A thick layer of dead cells in the epidermis provides a physical barrier to viruses, bacteria, and microbes. As the epidermis sheds, microbes are removed.
    - **Hair:** Hair within the nose filters microbes, dust, and pollutants from the air to prevent them from invading the body.
    - **Mucous membranes:** Mucous membranes produce mucus to trap microbes so they cannot spread to the rest of the body.
    - **Cilia:** Cilia line the upper respiratory tract and trap the microbes. They further propels the inhaled debris to the throat that is then expelled out of the body .
    - **Urine:** Urine flushes microbes out of the body via the urethra.
    - **Defecation and vomiting:** The body expels microorganisms via bowel movements and vomit.
  - **Chemical barriers** form another first line of defense against invading microbes.
    - **Acidity:** Skin acidity inhibits bacterial growth.
    - **Lysozyme:** Lysozyme is an enzyme that is secreted in tears, sweat, and saliva. It breaks down cell walls and acts as an antibiotic by killing bacteria.
    - **Saliva:** It dilutes the number of microorganisms in the body and washes the teeth and mouth.
    - **Gastric juice:** As the gastric juices contain acids, they destroy bacteria.
    - **Sebum:** Unsaturated fatty acids known as sebum provide a protective covering on the skin and inhibits growth.

- **Hyaluronic acid:** This is a gelatinous substance, and slows the spread of microorganisms that may harm the body.
- Second line of defense is nonspecific resistance and is part of innate immunity
  - Nonspecific resistance (innate immunity) The second line of defense of the immune system is the nonspecific resistance. These defense mechanisms destroy invaders in a general way and do not target specific antigens.
    - **Phagocytes:** Phagocytic cells ingest and destroy microbes that gains entry into body tissues.
    - **Inflammation:** Inflammation is a localized response in the tissue that occurs when tissues are damaged or in response to other stimuli. Inflammation occurs when white blood cells flood an area of invasion by microbes. The response includes swelling, redness, heat, and pain.
    - **Fever:** Fever inhibits bacterial growth and increases the rate of tissue repair during an infection in the body.
- The third line of defense is specific resistance, which is considered a function of acquired immunity.
  - Specific resistance (acquired immunity)
    - The final line of defense is specific resistance, which is a component of acquired immunity. Most antigens are proteins.

- Specific resistance depends on type of antigens that are found in foreign microbes.
- The antigens act as a stimulus to produce an immune response.
- **Lymphocytes:** Specific white blood cells, T cells and B cells, are responsible for acquired immunity. A specific immune response occurs when antibodies produced by B cells encounter antigens.

ROLE OF NURSES IN PREVENTION OF NOSOCOMIAL INFECTIONS

Nosocomial infections have deep effects on the patient in more than one way. The patient has to spend two and a half times more than a patient in normal conditions. The cost of treatment increases. Nurses can play a pivotal role in prevention of nosocomial infections. Nurse should be familiar with practices to prevent occurrence and spread of infection, including:

- Knowledge of proper techniques of catheter insertion and care
- Catheterizing only when necessary
- Emphasizing hand-washing
- Using aseptic technique for catheter insertion
- Securing catheter properly
- Maintaining closed sterile drainage
- Obtaining urine samples aseptically
- Maintaining unobstructed urine flow when dealing with a urinary tract infection patient.

Assess Yourself

LONG ANSWER QUESTIONS

1. What are portals of entry and exit of microbes?
2. What are the different modes of entry of microorganism into the body?
3. Explain the portals of exit in microorganisms.
4. Explain the portals and exit of microorganisms.
5. What is infection?
6. Explain the mode of transmission of infection.

SHORT NOTES

1. What is nosocomial infection
2. List few nosocomial infections

MULTIPLE CHOICE QUESTIONS

1. *Vibrio cholerae* contaminates:
   - a. Water
   - b. Air
   - c. Food
   - d. Soil

2. The most common cause of nosocomial infections is:
   - a. *Staphylococcus*
   - b. *E. coli*
   - c. *Acinetobacter*
   - d. *P. aeruginosa*

3. Gastroenteritis is caused by:
   - a. *Staphylococcus*
   - b. *Salmonella*
   - c. *Clostridium*
   - d. *Streptocccus*

4. Most common nosocomial infection is:
   - a. Surgical site infections
   - b. Urinary tract infections
   - c. Respiratory infections
   - d. Gastroenteritis

ANSWERS TO MCQS

1. a   **2.** c   **3.** c   **4.** b

Growth Factors

INTRODUCTION

Bacterial growth could be observed in two ways—increase in size of the individual cell and increase in the total number of cells. Increase in total number of cells can be observed by bacterial counts. The growth of the bacteria can be represented on a growth curve.

BACTERIAL GROWTH CURVE

Number of bacteria in the culture at different periods (**Figure 11.1**) may be represented as:

- Total count: It includes both living and dead bacteria.
- Viable count: It includes only the living bacteria.

Growth Phases

Lag Phase

In this phase, there is an increase in cell size but it does not multiply. Time is required for adaptation (synthesis of new enzymes) to new environment. During this phase, vigorous metabolic activities occur but cells do not divide.

Exponential Phase or Logarithmic (Log) Phase

The cells multiply at the maximum rate in this exponential phase, i.e. there is linear relationship between time and logarithm of the number of cells. Mass increases in an exponential manner. This continues until either one or more nutrients in the medium are exhausted, or toxic metabolic products accumulate and inhibit growth. The average time

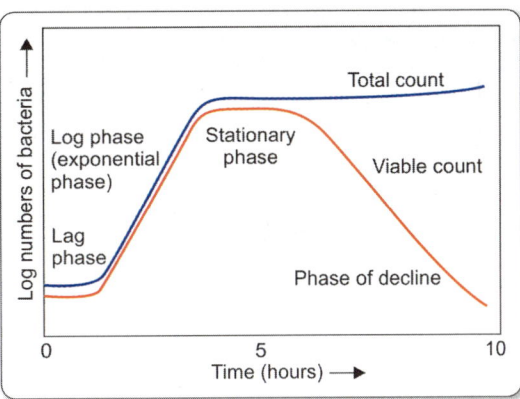

Figure 11.1: Bacterial growth curve

required for the population to double is known as the generation time or doubling time.

Maximal Stationary Phase

Due to exhaustion of nutrients or accumulation of toxic products, death of bacteria starts and the growth ceases completely. The count remains stationary due to balance between multiplication and death rate. Production of exotoxins and spore formation takes place in this phase.

Decline Phase or Death Phase

In this phase, there is progressive death of cells. However, some living bacteria use the breakdown products of dead bacteria as nutrient (saprophytic bacteria).

FACTORS AFFECTING BACTERIAL GROWTH

Temperature

Most bacteria are mesophilic. Mesophilic bacteria grow best at 30°–37°C. Optimum temperature for growth of common pathogenic bacteria is 37°C. Bacteria of a species will not grow but may remain alive at a maximum and a minimum temperature. Most bacteria are killed at 56°C in 30 minutes.

> **Also Know**
>
> Optimum temperature is the particular temperature range required by bacteria for their growth.

Terms to Learn

- **Psychrophilic**: Bacteria that grow at an optimum temperature of 10°–20°C
- **Mesophilic**: Bacteria tha grow at an optimum temperature of 20°–40°C
- **Thermophilic**: Bacteria that live best at the temperature of 50°–60°C.

pH of the Medium

Most pathogenic bacteria grow best in pH 7.2–7.4. *Vibrio cholerae* can grow in pH 8.2–9.0.

Carbon Dioxide

All bacteria require carbon dioxide for their growth. Most bacteria produce carbon dioxide.

Oxygen

Bacteria may be classified into four groups on oxygen requirement :

1. **Aerobes:** They cannot grow without oxygen, e.g. *Mycobacterium tuberculosis.*
2. **Facultative anaerobes:** These grow under both aerobic and anaerobic conditions. Most bacteria are facultative anaerobes, e.g. Enterobacteriaceae.
3. **Anaerobes:** They only grow in absence of free oxygen, e.g. *Clostridium*, Bacteroides.
4. **Microaerophils:** They grow best in oxygen less than that present in the air, e.g. *Campylobacter.*

Nutrients

Bacteria need nutrients for their growth and some need more nutrients than others. Bacteria normally feed on organic matter as well as material for cell formation. Organic matter also contains the necessary energy. Such matter must be soluble in water and must be of low molecular weight to be able to pass through the cell membrane.

> **Also Know**
>
> - Autotrophs live only on inorganic substances, i.e. do not require organic nutrients for growth. They are not of medical importance.
> - Heterotrophs require organic materials for growth, e.g., proteins, carbohydrates and lipids as source of energy.
> - Saprophytes grow on dead organic matter.

Relative Humidity

The content of water in the air is one of the major factors determining the ability to survive. At a very low humidity and high-temperature, cells face dehydration whereas high humidity may give cells protection against the solar radiation.

Assess Yourself

LONG ANSWER QUESTION

1. Write about factors influencing growth of microorganisms

MULTIPLE CHOICE QUESTIONS

1. Which of the following factor does not affect microbial growth?
   - a. Moisture
   - b. Disinfection
   - c. Darkness
   - d. Temperature

2. The typical bacterial growth curve shows:
   - a. 5 phases
   - b. 4 phases
   - c. 3 phases
   - d. 2 phases

3. Bacteria that grow at an optimum temperature of 20°–40°C are known as:
   - a. Thermophilic
   - b. Mesophilic
   - c. Psychrophilic
   - d. None

4. *Vibrio cholerae* can grow in pH of:
   - a. 7.2–7.4
   - b. 7.4–7.6
   - c. 8.4–9.2
   - d. 8.2–9.0

5. Saprophytes grow on:
   - a. Dead organic matter
   - b. Inorganic substances
   - c. Organic material
   - d. None of the above

ANSWERS TO MCQs

1. c **2.** b **3.** b **4.** d **5.** a

Collection of Specimens

INTRODUCTION

The proper collection and transport of patient's specimens for culture is the most important step in the recovery of pathogenic organisms responsible for infectious disease. A poorly collected specimen may lead to failure to isolate the causative organism(s) and/or result in recovery and subsequent treatment of contaminating organisms.

BASIC INSTRUCTIONS FOR SPECIMEN COLLECTION

- Collect the specimen from the actual site of infection. Avoid contamination from adjacent tissue or fluids.
- Collect the specimen at the optimal time. For example, collect sputum for culture in the early morning.
- Collect a sufficient quantity of material.
- Use appropriate collection devices such as sterile, leak-proof containers. Use appropriate transport media.
- Whenever possible, collect the specimen prior to the administration of antibiotics.

- Properly label the specimen with two patient identifiers (complete name and medical record number or date of birth) as well as the specific source of the specimen.
- Minimize transport time and ensure that the transport environment is appropriate
- Submission of a tissue biopsy is preferable to swabbing the area and submitting a swab for culture.

STOOL SPECIMENS

The stool specimen can be obtained by one of the following methods:
- Pass stool directly into a sterile, wide-mouth, leak-proof container with a tight fitting lid.
- Pass stool into a clean, dry bedpan, and transfer into a sterile leak proof container with a tight fitting lid.
- Keep stool specimen cool.
- Do not incubate.
- Do not use toilet paper to collect stool. Toilet paper may contain substances, which are inhibitory for some fecal pathogens.
- Stool for ova and parasites should be placed in preservative immediately after collection.

RECTAL SWABS

- Pass the tip of a sterile swab approximately 1 inch beyond the anal sphincter.
- Carefully rotate the swab to sample the anal crypts and withdraw the swab. Place the swab in transport medium.

THROAT SWABS

- Do not obtain throat sample if epiglottis is inflamed, as sampling may cause serious respiratory obstruction.
- Depress tongue gently with tongue depressor.
- Extend sterile swab between the tonsillar pillars and behind the uvula.
- Avoid touching the cheeks, tongue, uvula or lips.
- To obtain sample, sweep the swab back and forth across the posterior pharynx, tonsillar areas and in particular any inflamed or ulcerated areas.

URINE SPECIMEN

General Considerations

- Never collect urine from a bedpan or urinal.
- Thoroughly clean the urethral opening (and vaginal vestibule in females) prior to collection procedures to ensure that the specimen obtained is not contaminated with colonizing microorganisms in this area. Use soap rather than disinfectants for cleaning the urethral area. If disinfectants are introduced into the urine during collection, they can inhibit the growth of microorganisms.
- Transport the specimen to the laboratory such that it will be plated within two hours of collection. Urine from clinics outside the main hospital campus should be place in tubes with preservative.
- These specimens can be held for eight hours. Alternatively, urine can be refrigerated for 24 hours before plating.
- Use sterile tubes or cups to collect and transport the urine.

Urine Specimen Collection (Female)

- The person obtaining the urine specimen should wash hands with soap and water, rinse and dry. If

the patient is collecting the specimen, she should be given detailed instructions.
- Cleanse the urethral opening and vaginal vestibule area with soapy water or clean gauze pads soaked with liquid soap.
- Rinse the area well with water or wet gauze pads.
- Hold labia apart during voiding. Allow a few milliliters to pass.
- Collect the midstream portion of urine in a sterile container.

Urine Specimen Collection (Male)

The person obtaining the specimen should wash their hands with soap and water, rinse and dry. If the patient is collecting the specimen, he should be given detailed instructions. Cleanse the penis, retract the foreskin (if not circumcised), and wash with soapy water. Rinse the area well with water. Keeping foreskin retracted; allow a few milliliters of urine to pass. Collect the midstream portion of urine in a sterile container.

BLOOD SPECIMEN

Venipuncture Procedure

- Position the patient in a chair, or sitting or lying on a bed.
- Select a suitable site for venipuncture, by placing the tourniquet 3–4 inches above the selected puncture site on the patient.
- Do not put the tourniquet on too tightly or leave it on the patient longer than 1 minute.
- Next, put on non-latex gloves, and palpate for a vein.
- When a vein is selected, cleanse the area in a circular motion, beginning at the site and working outward. Allow the area to air dry.
- After the area is cleansed, it should not be touched or palpated again. If you find it necessary to reevaluate the site by palpation, the area needs to be re-cleansed before the venipuncture is performed.
- Ask the patient to make a fist; avoid "pumping the fist."
- Grasp the patient's arm firmly using your thumb to draw the skin taut and anchor the vein.
- Swiftly insert the needle through the skin into the lumen of the vein.

- The needle should form a 15°–30° angle with the arm surface. Avoid excess probing.
- When the last tube is filling, remove the tourniquet.
- Remove the needle from the patient's arm using a swift backward motion.
- Place gauze immediately on the puncture site. Apply and hold adequate pressure to avoid formation of a hematoma.
- After holding pressure for 1–2 minutes, tape a fresh piece of gauze or band-aid to the puncture site.

Fingerstick Procedure

- The best locations for fingersticks are the 3rd (middle) and 4th (ring) fingers of the non-dominant hand.
- Avoid puncturing a finger that is cold or cyanotic, swollen, scarred, or covered with a rash.

- When a site is selected, put on gloves, and cleanse the selected puncture area.
- Massage the finger toward the selected site prior to the puncture.
- Using a sterile safety lancet, make a skin puncture just off the center of the finger pad.
- The puncture should be made perpendicular to the ridges of the fingerprint so that the drop of blood does not run down the ridges.
- Wipe away the first drop of blood, which tends to contain excess tissue fluid.
- Collect drops of blood into the collection tube/ device by gentle pressure on the finger.
- Avoid excessive pressure or "milking" that may squeeze tissue fluid into the drop of blood.
- Cap, rotate and invert the collection device to mix the blood collected.
- Have the patient hold a small gauze pad over the puncture site for a few minutes to stop the bleeding.

 **Assess Yourself**

LONG ANSWER QUESTIONS

1. Collection of specimen.
2. What is venipuncture? Discuss its procedure.

MULTIPLE CHOICE QUESTIONS

1. Sputum specimen should be taken preferably in:
   a. Afternoon
   b. Early morning
   c. Evening
   d. Late afternoon

2. The following statements are true except:
   a. Urine sample should be collected from bedpan
   b. Hands should be washed before taking urine sample
   c. Midstream portion of urine should be taken
   d. Soap should be used to cleanse the urethral area

3. Torniquet during venipuncture should be placed:
   a. 3–4 inches above punctured site
   b. 7–8 inches below punctured site
   c. Just above the punctured site
   d. An inch above the punctured site

4. The best site for fingerstick procedure:
   a. First finger of dominant hand
   b. Fourth finger of dominant hand
   c. First finger of non dominant hand
   d. Fourth finger of non dominant hand

ANSWERS TO MCQs

1. b 2. a 3. a 4. d

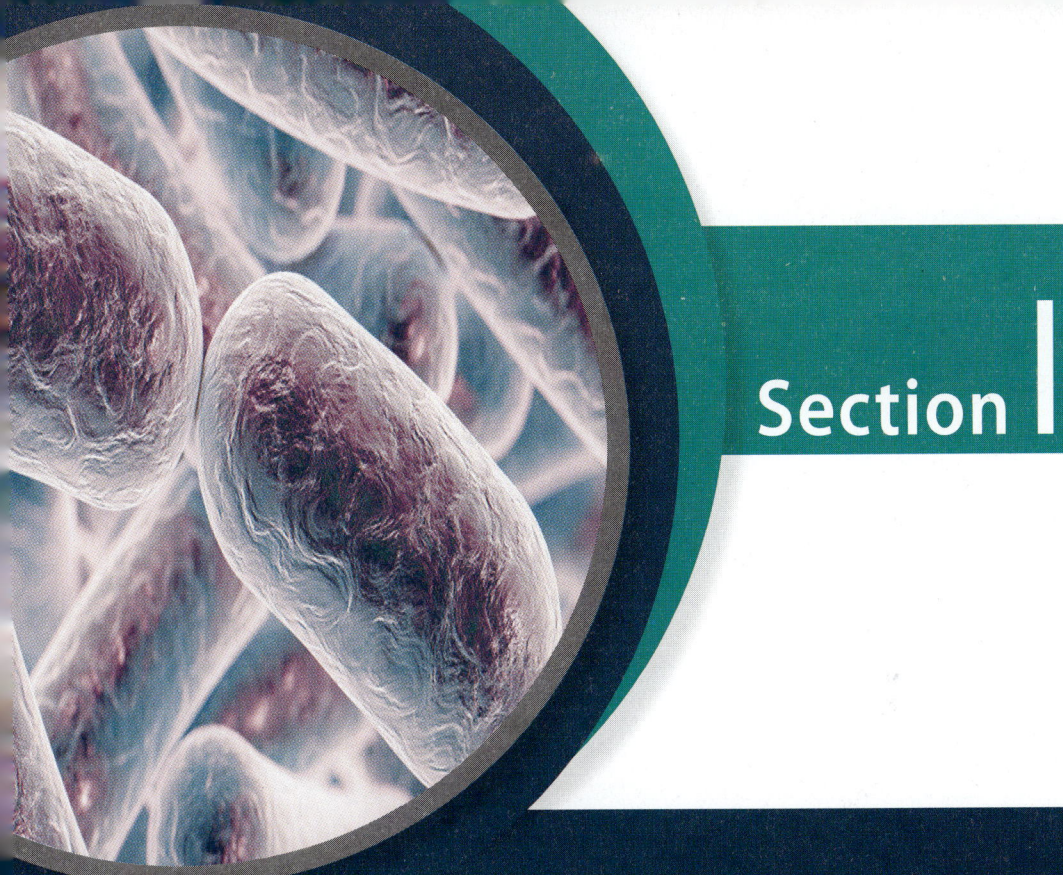

Section IV

IMMUNOLOGY

Basics of Immunology
(Including National Immunization Schedule)

INTRODUCTION

Our body is under threat constantly by various factors like pathogenic organisms, toxins, carcinogens etc. To protect our body from these harmful factors, the defense system of the body comes into play. This defense system is also known as immune system of the body. Immunity is defined as the resistance of the body towards the harmful effects caused by the pathogenic organisms and other toxic factors. Immunity is of two types as shown in **Figure 13.1**:

1. Innate immunity
2. Acquired immunity

INNATE IMMUNITY

Innate means *inborn or natural*. This is the type of immunity, which is present since birth and is

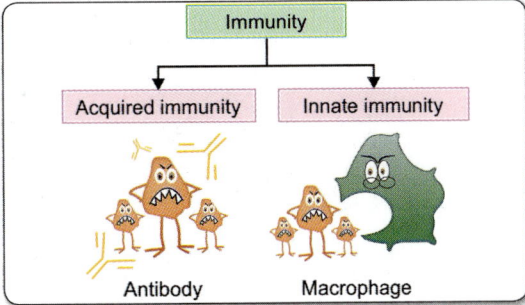

Figure 13.1: Types of immunity

possessed by an individual due to his genetic and constitutional make up. It can be nonspecific, if the resistance is against infections in general or specific, if the resistance is against a particular organism or toxin. It is considered at three levels.

1. **Species immunity:** It is the resistance shown by all members of a species. For example, Guinea pigs and humans are prone to tuberculosis, while dogs, sheep and horses are immune to it.

2. **Racial immunity:** The resistance to infection also varies amongst various races within a species. These are known to be genetic in origin. For example, black races in humans are more susceptible to tuberculosis as compared to white races.

3. **Individual immunity**: Individual immunity is the susceptibility of different individuals in a race towards an infection. For example, if a large number of people are exposed to a particular infection, some won't be affected by it, some will develop a mild infection and others will develop the infection severely.

Mechanisms of Innate Immunity

Epithelial Surfaces

- **Skin:** Skin acts as a mechanical barrier for the microorganisms to enter the body. The high concentration of salt in drying sweat, sebaceous secretions and long chain fatty acids act as bactericidal agents as well.

- **Respiratory tract:** The mucus secretion of respiratory tract traps the inhaled particles and hair-like cilia propel the particles towards the pharynx, initiating the cough reflex. The cough reflex acts as a defense mechanism.

- **Gastrointestinal tract:** The enzymatic activity in saliva and the acidic pH of gastric juices destroy many microorganisms.

- **Conjunctiva:** Lysozyme present in tears acts as bactericidal agent. Tears also help in flushing away microorganisms and other dust particles.

- **Genitourinary tract:** Urine with its flushing action helps in eliminating bacteria from urethra. Acidic pH of vaginal secretions in females renders vagina free of many pathogens.

Complement System of the Body

Complement system plays an important role in destroying the pathogenic bacteria entering blood and tissues.

Phagocytosis by Neutrophils and Macrophages (Figure 13.2)

With the release of chemicals like histamine from damaged body cells, neutrophils and macrophages concentrate at the sites of infection. The cellular extensions, pseudopodia, surround the pathogen and engulf it forming an internal vesicle. The vesicle then fuses with the lysosome to digest the pathogen.

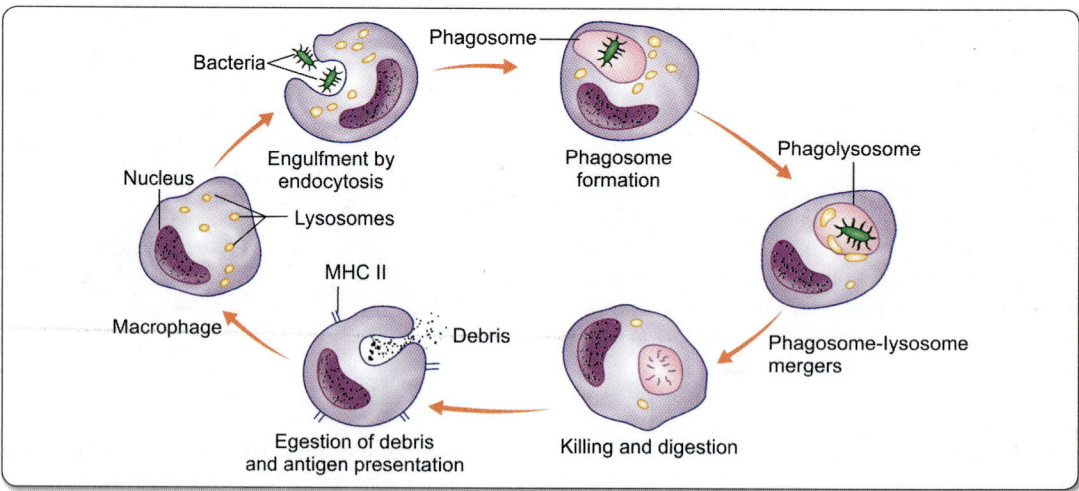

Figure 13.2: Stages of phagocytosis

Abbreviation: MHC, major histocompatibility complex

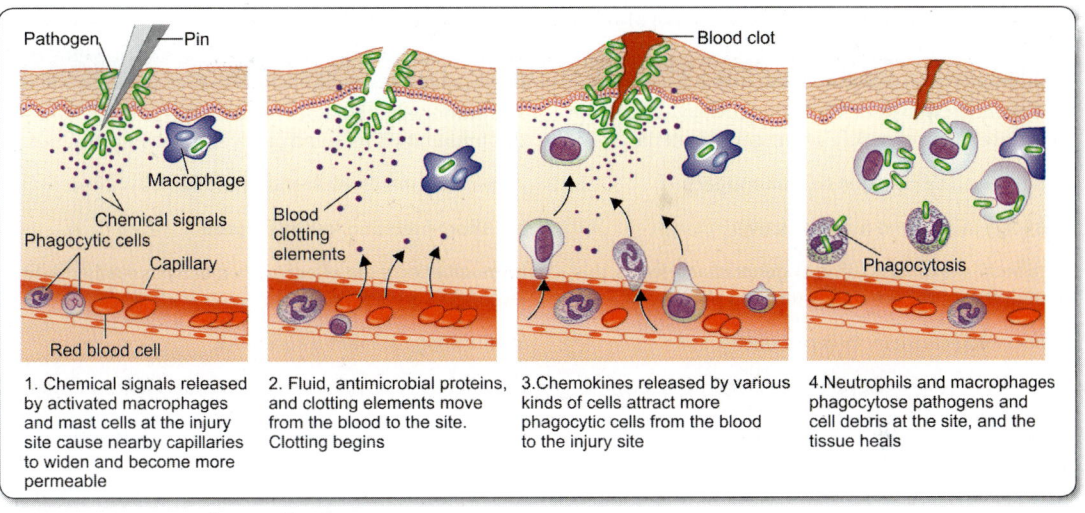

1. Chemical signals released by activated macrophages and mast cells at the injury site cause nearby capillaries to widen and become more permeable

2. Fluid, antimicrobial proteins, and clotting elements move from the blood to the site. Clotting begins

3. Chemokines released by various kinds of cells attract more phagocytic cells from the blood to the injury site

4. Neutrophils and macrophages phagocytose pathogens and cell debris at the site, and the tissue heals

Figure 13.3: Stages of wound healing

Inflammation

With the tissue damage, mast cells release histamine that leads to local vasodilatation and increased capillary permeability. The chemotactic factors thus released, recruit wandering macrophages to the site of damage **(Figure 13.3)**. Inflammation is necessary to allow immune cell to access infected tissues. The four signs of inflammation are:

1. Redness
2. Swelling
3. Heat
4. Pain

Fever

Rise in temperature or fever is a physiological response of the body that helps in accelerating the physiological processes and hence, causes destruction of microorganisms.

ACQUIRED IMMUNITY

An individual also acquires the resistance to fight against the microorganisms during his lifetime and this is called acquired immunity. It is of two types:

1. Active immunity
2. Passive immunity.

Active Immunity

It is induced by an infection or by contact with antigens. It can be either natural (produced due to clinical or subclinical infection) or artificial (induced by vaccination).

- **Natural active immunity:** It is resistance developed from clinical or subclinical infections.
  - **Long-lasting immunity:** Diphtheria, measles, mumps, whooping cough
  - **Short-time immunity:** Influenza and common cold.
- **Artificial active immunity:** This is the resistance that is induced by vaccines in the body. Vaccines are prepared from live, attenuated or killed microorganisms, or their antigens and toxins.
  - **Bacterial vaccines:**
    - Live: Ty21a for typhoid, Bacillus Calmette Güerin (BCG) for tuberculosis
    - Killed: Cholera, pertussis, TAB for enteric fever
  - **Bacterial products:** Tetanus, diphtheria toxoid
  - **Viral vaccines:**
    - **Live:** Sabin vaccine for polio, MMR for mumps, measles and rubella
    - **Killed:** Salk vaccine for polio, hepatitis B vaccine.

TABLE 13.1: Differences between Active and Passive Immunity

Active immunity	Passive immunity
The immune system of the body actively takes part in response to the exposure of antigenic material	The immune system does not actively participates and this immunity is received passively by the host
It is induced by infection or immunogens	Administration of ready-made antibodies is done
It is long-lasting and more effective	It is short-lived and less efficacious
Antibodies take some time in generation. Hence, this immunity is effective only after a lag period	Immunity comes in effect immediately as ready-made antibodies are administered
Immunological memory is present	Immunological memory is absent
It is not effective and applicable in immunodeficient persons	It is effective and applicable in immunodeficient persons

Also Know

In killed vaccines, the organisms are killed by heat, formalin, alcohol and phenol. Toxoids are prepared from inactivating the bacterial exotoxins by formalin or alum. Toxoids are immunogenic and are not toxigenic.

Mechanisms of Active Immunity

Active immunity stimulates both humoral and cell-mediated immunity.

- **Humoral immunity**: Humoral immunity or antibody-mediated immunity depends on the synthesis of antibodies by plasma cells. The specific antibodies, thus produced, combine with specific antigens and modify their activity.
- **Cell-mediated immunity**: The cell-mediated immunity (by sensitized T-lymphocytes) is important in resistance to chronic bacterial infections.

Passive Immunity

In passive immunity, the immune system of the individual plays no active role. Readymade antibodies are transferred into the individual. It is short-lived and is useful when immunity is required immediately. It is of two types:

1. **Natural:** It includes transfer of maternal antibodies (IgG) transplacentally to the fetus and to the infant through milk. It provides immediate protection to the infant/fetus and protects them till their own immune system matures.

2. **Artificial:** Parenteral administration of antibodies in done in this type of passive immunity. The agents used are hyperimmune sera of animal or human origin, convalescent sera and pooled human gamma globulin.

The difference between active and passive immunity are summarized in **Table 13.1**.

Also Know

Passive immunity is also induced for suppression of active immunity. For example, in Rh negative mothers with Rh positive babies, Rh immunoglobulin is induced during delivery to prevent immune response to Rh factor.

Terms to Learn

- **Combined immunization:** A combination of active and passive immunization is employed simultaneously in this case. Passive immunity provides protection till the active immunity becomes effective.
- **Herd immunity:** The overall resistance in a community is called herd immunity. If herd immunity is low, outbreaks of epidemics increase on introduction of a suitable pathogen.

ANTIGEN

An antigen is a substance, which stimulates the production of a specific antibody, after it enters the body.

Types of Antigen

Antigens are of two types:

1. **Complete antigen:** These can induce antibody formation by themselves and can react specifically with these antibodies.
2. **Haptens:** These cannot induce antibody formation, but after covalently linking to a carrier protein, it is capable of inducing antibody formation.

> *Also Know*
>
> The smallest unit of antigenicity is called *epitope* or *antigenic determinant*. They have a specific chemical structure, electrical charge and induce a specific antibody formation, which reacts at that site.

Properties of Antigens

- **Foreignness:** In order to induce an immune response, an antigen should be foreign to the body.
- **Size:** Larger the molecular size of the antigen, higher is the antigenicity.
- **Chemical nature:** Out of the 4 major biomolecules, proteins are more effective antigens.
- **Species specificity:** Tissues of all individuals in a species contain species-specific antigens. It plays an important role in evolutionary relationship.
- **Isospecificity:** Isoantigens are found only in some members of a species. This helps in grouping of the species according to the presence of an isoantigen. Blood grouping is one example depending on human erythrocyte antigens.
- **Autospecificity:** Auto means *self*. Autospecific antigens are generally nonantigenic.
- **Organ specificity:** The organ specific antigens are confined to a particular organ. Organs like lens protein, brain and kidney of one species share specificity with that of another species.
- **Heterogenic specificity:** Some closely related antigens are found in different biological species like bacteria, plants and animals. These are called heterogenic or heterophile antigens.

> *Also Know*
>
> Heterophile antigens are used for serological diagnosis of several diseases.

ANTIBODY

Antibody or immunoglobulin is a substance produced in the body in response to an antigen and reacts with it specifically.

Structure of Immunoglobulin

Immunoglobulins are glycoprotein in nature and each molecule consists of two identical heavy (H) chains that are longer in size and two identical light (L) chains that are shorter in size. The 2 H chains are joined by 1–5 disulfide bonds and the L and H chains are joined by disulfide bonds **(Figure 13.4)**. The H chains are structurally and antigenically different for each class of immunoglobulins. There are five classes of immunoglobulins namely, IgG, IgM, IgA, IgD and IgE.

> *Also Know*
>
> The five classes of immunoglobulins, IgG, IgM, IgA, IgD and IgE are designated depending on presence of heavy chain gamma (γ), mu (μ), alpha (α), delta (δ) and epsilon (ε), respectively.

Light chains are similar in all classes. They occur in two forms: kappa (κ) and lambda (λ). An immunoglobulin has either 2 kappa or 2 lambda chains, but never both.

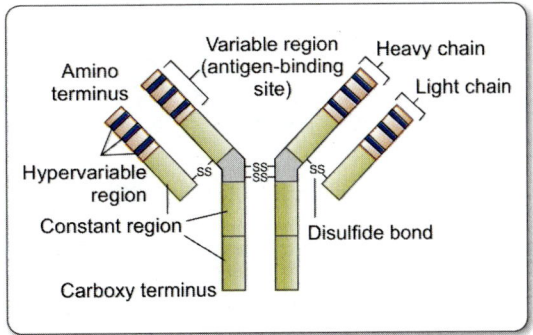

Figure 13.4: Structure of immunoglobulin

Section IV • Immunology

TABLE 13.2: Properties of Immunoglobulins

Property	IgG	IgA	IgM	IgD	IgE
Molecular weight	150,000	160,000	900,000	180,000	190,000
Heavy chain	γ	α	μ	δ	ε
Serum conc. (mg/mL)	12	2	1.2	0.03	0.0004
Half-life (days)	23	6–8	5	3	2–3
Placental transport	Present	Absent	Absent	Absent	Absent
Present in mother's milk	Present	Present	Absent	Absent	Absent
Heat stability	Yes	Yes	Yes	Yes	No

The site for combining with antigen is composed of both H and L chains. This part has a constant region called carboxy terminus and other variable terminal is called amino terminus.

Types of Immunoglobulins

Few important properties of various immunoglobulins are summarized in **Table 13.2**.

IgG

It is the major serum immunoglobulin and constitutes about 80% of all immunoglobulins **(Figure 13.5)**. It is the only antibody that passes through the placenta. It is involved in complement activation and phagocytosis and protects against the microorganisms, which are active in blood and tissues.

IgA

It is the second most abundant class of immunoglobulins and constitutes about 10–13% of total serum immunoglobulins. It is a principal immunoglobulin present in milk, saliva, tears, sweat, nasal fluids, and colostrum and in secretions of respiratory, intestinal and genital system. Initially it is a monomer and it attains a secretory component later. It becomes dimer linked by J-chains and is known as secretory IgA **(Figure 13.6)**.

IgM

IgM is the largest antibody and the first immunoglobulin that is produced on exposure. It is the third most abundant immunoglobulin. It is responsible for complement activation and forms ABO antibodies. It is a pentamer **(Figure 13.7)**.

Also Know

The molecular wt. of IgM is 900,000–1,000,000 and hence, it is called a millionaire molecule.

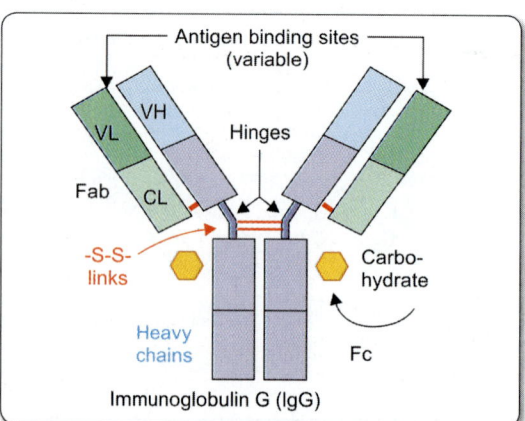

Figure 13.5: Structure of IgG

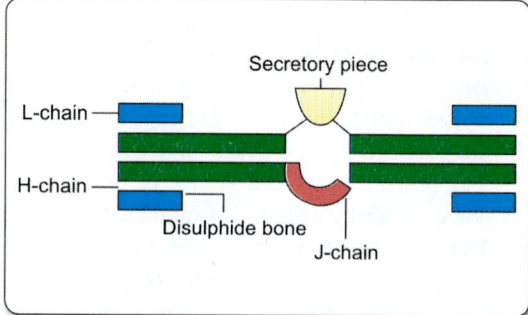

Figure 13.6: Structure of secretory IgA molecule

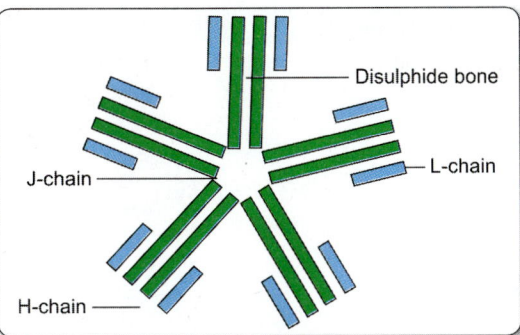

Figure 13.7: Structure of IgM molecule

(Labels: Disulphide bone, L-chain, J-chain, H-chain)

IgD

It is a monomer and is similar to IgG in structure. It is short-lived and plays an important role in secondary immune response. It occurs in combination with IgM on surface of B lymphocytes and is involved in antigen recognition by B cells.

IgE

It is extravascular in distribution and is a monomer. It is responsible in the release of histamine from basophil and mast cells and hence, it is involved in anaphylactic type of hypersensitivity. It is produced by respiratory and intestinal tract linings. It is increased in atopic allergy and parasitic infestations.

CELLS OF IMMUNE SYSTEM

The various cells along with their functions have been summarized in **Table 13.3**.

Also Know

Specific tissue macrophages are as follows:
- Liver: Kupffer cells
- **Lung:** Alveolar macrophages
- **Connective tissue:** Histiocytes
- **Bone:** Osteoclasts
- **Brain:** Microglial cells.

Section IV • Immunology

TABLE 13.3: Characteristics of Cells of Immune System

Cell type	Characteristics	Image
T-lymphocytes	Mature in thymus; possess T-cell receptor; responsible for cell-mediated immunity; three types of T lymphocytes: 1. **T-helper (T$_H$) cells:** Recognize and interact with antigen 2. **T-suppressor (T$_S$) cells:** Suppress cell-mediated and humoral immunity 3. **Cytotoxic T (T$_C$) cells:** Activated under influence of cytokines	
B-lymphocytes	Mature in bone marrow; contain unique IgM receptor; responsible for humoral immunity; after activation, divides into two types: 1. **Memory B cells:** Express membrane bound antibody 2. **Effector B cells or plasma cells:** Produce antibodies	
Natural killer cells	Kills tumor cells and virus-infected cells; action is independent of antibody; activity does not require sensitization by prior antigenic contact	

Contd...

Cell type	Characteristics	Image
Monocytes	Stored in spleen; differentiates into macrophages and dendritic cells in response to inflammation	
Macrophages	Phagocytic cell that consumes foreign pathogens and cancer cells; stimulates response of other immune cells	
Neutrophils	First to respond at the site of infection or trauma; most abundant of all leukocytes; causes release of toxins that kill or inhibit bacteria or fungi	
Eosinophils	Less phagocytic than neutrophils; found in large numbers in allergic inflammation and parasitic infections	
Basophils	Present in blood and tissues; responsible for defense against parasites; releases histamines that cause inflammation and may be responsible for allergic reactions	
Mast cells	Present in connective tissues and mucous membranes; dilates blood vessels and induces inflammation through release of histamine and heparin; involved in wound healing and defense against pathogens	

Contd...

Cell type	Characteristics	Image
Dendritic cells	Present in epithelial tissues including skin, lung and gastrointestinal tract; presents antigen on its surface, thereby triggering adaptive immunity	

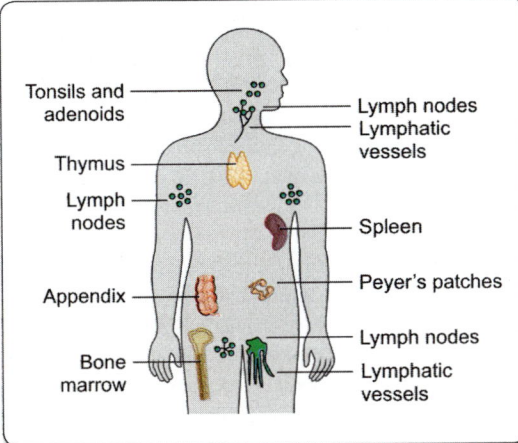

Figure 13.8: Organs of immune system

ORGANS OF IMMUNE SYSTEM

The important organs of the immune system (**Figure 13.8**) have been described below.

Thymus

- Greyish, flat, bilobed lymphoid organ present in the upper part of chest cavity
- Primary function is to produce T lymphocytes
- Grows in size till puberty and later regresses in size
- Precursors of T lymphocytes are present in cortex; they pass to medulla after maturation. From medulla, they migrate to secondary lymphoid organs.

Bone Marrow

- Site of origin of B Lymphocytes
- Equivalent to bursa of Fabricius in birds

Lymph Nodes

- Small bean-shaped clusters present along the course of lymphatic vessels
- Act as filters of lymph
- Lymphocytes, macrophages and dendritic cells are arranged in follicles in the cortex area.

Spleen

- Largest lymphoid organ
- Traps blood-borne antigens
- Red pulp is rich in red blood cells and macrophages and white pulp contains primary and secondary lymphoid follicles having B-lymphocytes.

Mucosa-associated Lymphoid Tissue

- Includes Peyer's patches of small intestine, tonsils, appendix, salivary glands, lacrimal glands and follicles in respiratory tract
- Present diffusely in submucosa and mucosa
- Contains both T and B lymphocytes.

Also Know

- Polio vaccines must be stored at minus 20°C.
- Typhoid, Diphtheria and tetanus toxoids (DT), DPT, BCG and tetanus vaccines should never be freeze dried.

IMMUNOPROPHYLAXIS

It is the prevention of disease by the production of active or passive immunity. Vaccination is used for this purpose by using vaccines, antisera or immune serum globulin (human).

Difference between Vaccine and Sera

Vaccine therapy for prevention or cure of infection has for its object the production of an active immunity to the specific bacteria concerned, while serum therapy produces a passive immunity only.

Know it ....

Cold Chain

Cold chain is a system of storing and transporting vaccines at a low temperature, ideally recommended for the vaccines. Maintenance of cold storage is important as vaccines may lose their potency if not properly stored at right temperature. All vaccines must be stored between 2° and 8°C.

Vaccination

- Immunity against pathogens (viruses and bacteria) is obtained by using: live attenuated, killed or altered antigens that stimulate the body to produce antibodies.
- Vaccines work with the immune system's ability to recognize and destroy foreign proteins (antigens).
- Vaccination prevents and control such diseases as cholera, rabies, poliomyelitis, diphtheria, tetanus, measles, and typhoid fever.

Vaccines

- Vaccines can be:
  - Prophylactic (e.g. to prevent or ameliorate the effects of a future infection by any natural or "wild" pathogen.
  - Therapeutic (e.g. vaccines against cancer that are still under investigation).

Types of Vaccines

- **Killed vaccines:** Virulent bacteria or viruses used to prepare these vaccines may be killed by heat (60°C) or by chemicals (formalin, phenol or merthiolate), for examples:
  - TAB vaccine against enteric fever (heat)
  - Salk vaccine against poliomyelitis (formalin)
  - Semple's vaccine against rabies (phenol)
  - Pertussis vaccine against whooping cough (merthiolate)
    Characteristics of killed vaccine:
    - Do not stimulate local immunity
    - Short lasting

- Do not stimulate cytotoxic T cell response in contrast to live attenuated vaccines
- Safe can be given to pregnant woman and immunocompromised host
- It is heat stable

- **Live attenuated vaccines:** Living microorganism loses its virulence so does not produce disease but produces immunity. It stimulates both humoral and cell mediated immunity, local and systemic. It is not given to pregnant women and immunocompromised hosts (may cause diseases). It is heat labile.
  It is prepared by:
  - Repeated subculture in unsuitable condition (chemical or media), e.g. BCG vaccine against T.B. and 17 D vaccine against yellow fever.
  - Growing at high temperature (Above optimum temp), e.g. Pasteur anthrax vaccine
  - Selection of mutant strains of low virulence, e.g., Sabin vaccine against poliomyelitis.
- Toxoids: It is prepared by detoxifying bacterial toxins. Bacterial exotoxins are treated by formalin to destroy toxicity and retain antigenicity, e.g., diphtheria and tetanus toxoid.
- Microbial products vaccines are prepared from bacterial products or viral components, e.g., Capsular polysaccharide vaccines are:
  - Poor immunogen in children below 2 years age, e.g., *H. influenzae* do not respond to T cell independent antigens in spite of its generation of IgM
  - Produce anticapsular opsonizing antibodies, for examples meningococci, pneumococci and *H. influenzae*
  - Cellular purified proteins of pertussis
  - Purified surface Ag of hepatitis B virus
  - Influenza viruses
    Prepared by recombinant DNA technology for improvement vaccines, e.g.
    - Subunit vaccines in which microbial polypeptides are isolated from the infective material hepatitis B and influenza viruses
    - Recombinant DNA-derived antigen vaccines in which Ag are synthesizing

by inserting the coding genes into *E. coli* or yeast cell as HBV vaccines

♦ Recombinant DNA avirulent vector vaccines in which the genes coding for the Ag is inserted into genome of an avirulent vector such as BCG vaccine

♦ **Synthetic peptide vaccines:** Synthesis of short peptides that correspond to antigenic determinants on a viral or bacterial proteins, e.g cholera toxins and poliovirus to produce Ab response.

IMMUNIZATION

Immunization is the process by which resistance to an infection is either induced or enhanced. The primary purpose of immunization is to prevent, control and eradicate various infections. Immunization can be achieved by vaccines. Vaccines are prepared from live, attenuated or killed microorganisms, or their antigens and toxins and are used to induce active immunity to an infectious agent. Examples of commonly used vaccines are as follows.

- **Bacterial vaccines:**
  - **Live:** Ty21a for typhoid, BCG for tuberculosis
  - **Killed:** Cholera, pertussis, TAB for enteric fever
- **Bacterial products:** Tetanus, diphtheria toxoid
- **Viral vaccines:**
  - Live: Sabin vaccine for polio, MMR for mumps, measles and rubella
  - Killed: Salk vaccine for polio, hepatitis B vaccine
- **Combined vaccines:** Diphtheria, pertussis (DPT), MMR

Combined Immunization (Vaccination)

Immunization against diseases is recommended in combination (for young children) as:

- Diphtheria, tetanus (lockjaw), and pertussis (whooping cough), given together (DTP).
- Measles, mumps, and rubella, give together as MMR
- Haemophilus influenzae b (Hib) with DTP
- Influenzae b (Hib) with inactivated poliomyelitis vaccine (IPV)
- Influenza and *Neisseria meningitides* (Meningococcal meningitis).

National Immunization Schedule (Table 13.4)

TABLE 13.4: National Immunization Schedule for Infants, Children and Pregnant Women

For Pregnant Women					
Vaccine	**When to give**	**Dose**	**Diluent**	**Route**	**Site**
TT-1	Early in pregnancy	0.5 mL	No	Intramuscular	Upper arm
TT-2	4 weeks after TT-1	0.5 mL	No	Intramuscular	Upper arm
TT-Booster	If received TT doses in a pregnancy within last 3 years	0.5 mL	No	Intramuscular	Upper arm

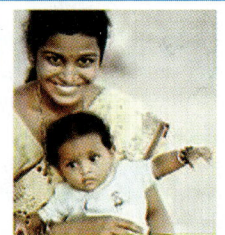

For Infants						
Vaccine	**When to give**	**Max. Age**	**Dose**	**Diluent**	**Route**	**Site**
BCG	At birth as early as possible	Till 1 year of age	0.1 mL (0.05 mL until 1 month age)	Sodium chloride	Intradermal	Left upper arm
Hepatitis B birth dose	At birth as early as possible	Within 24 hours	0.5 mL	NO	Intramuscular	Anterolateral side of mid-thigh LEFT

Contd...

Section IV • Immunology

OPV-0	At birth as early as possible	Within the first 15 days	2 drops	NO	Oral	
OPV 1, 2 & 3	At 6, 10 and 14 weeks	Till 5 years of age	2 drops	NO	Oral	
Rota virus vaccine	At 6, 10 and 14 weeks	Till 1 year of age	5 drops	NO	Oral	
IPV (inactivated polio vaccine)	At 6 and 14 weeks	Up to 1 year of age	0.1 mL	NO	Intradermal	Right upper arm
Pentavalent 1, 2 and 3	At 6, 10 and 14 weeks	Till 1 year of age	0.5 mL	NO	Intramuscular	Anterolateral side of mid-thigh LEFT
Measles 1st dose	9–12 completed months	Given till 5 years of age	0.5 mL	Sterile water	Subcutaneous	Right upper arm
Japanese Encephalitis 1st dose	9–12 completed months	Till 15 years	0.5 mL	Phosphate buffer	Subcutaneous	Left upper arm
Vitamin A (1st dose)	At 9 completed months with measles	Till 5 years of age	1 mL (1 lakh IU)	NO	Oral	
For Children						
DTP Booster –1	16–24 months	7 years	0.5 mL	NO	Intramuscular	Anterolateral side of mid-thigh LEFT
Measles 2nd dose	16–24 months	Till 5 years of age	0.5 mL	Sterile water	Subcutaneous	Right upper arm
OPV Booster	16–24 months	Till 5 years of age	2 drops	NO	Oral	
Japanese Encephalitis 2nd dose	16–24 months		0.5 mL	Phosphate buffer	Subcutaneous	Left upper arm
Vitamin A (2nd to 9th dose)	16 months. Then, 1 dose every 6 months	Till 5 years of age	2 mL (2 lakh IU)	NO	Oral	
DPT Booster –2	5–6 years	7 years	0.5 mL	NO	Intramuscular	Upper arm (Left)
TT	10 years and 16 years		0.5 mL	NO	Intramuscular	Upper arm

Note:
- Give TT-2 or Booster doses before 36 weeks of pregnancy. However, give these even if more than 36 weeks have passed. Give TT to a woman in labour, if she has not previously received TT.
- JE Vaccine, in select endemic districts after the campaign.
- The 2nd to 9th doses of Vitamin A can be administered to children 1-5 years old during biannual rounds, in collaboration with ICDS.

HYPERSENSITIVITY AND AUTOIMMUNITY

Hypersensitivity

Although immune responses are meant to protect our body, sometimes they might cause excessive reactions which leads to damage of the tissues, development of some disease or even death in a sensitized host. Such a reaction is called hypersensitivity reaction. They are either "immediate" i.e. reaction appears quickly and "delayed" i.e. reactions appear slowly in 24–72 hours. Coomb and Gel gave the classification of hypersensitivity reactions in 1963 and divided it in four major types that are summarized in **Table 13.5**.

Autoimmunity

Our immune system has been developed in a way that it recognizes difference between the cells of the body and foreign substances. Autoimmunity can be defined as a condition in which our immune system reacts against body's own cells by making antibodies. This leads to functional and structural damage to the tissues. The diseases produced as a result of such a reaction are called autoimmune diseases. Common examples of autoimmune diseases are, systemic lupus erythematosus (SLE), rheumatoid arthritis (RA), multiple sclerosis, type 1 diabetes mellitus, Grave's disease, myasthenia gravis, etc.

TABLE 13.5: Four Major Types of Hypersensitivity Reactions (Coomb and Gel)

Type	Name	Mechanism	Disease examples
Type I	Immediate hypersensitivity	IgE-mediated degranulation of mast cells following antigen binding and cross-linking of IgE	Allergic asthma, allergic rhinitis, anaphylaxis
Type II	Antibody-mediated hypersensitivity	IgM/IgG antibody: antigen interactions on target cell surfaces	Drug-induced thrombocytopenia, myasthenia gravis, Graves disease, hemolytic anemia of newborn
Type III	Immune complex-mediated hypersensitivity	Immune complex formation and deposition in tissues leading to local or systemic inflammatory reactions	Rheumatoid arthritis, systemic lupus erythematosus (SLE), Good Pasture's syndrome, arthus reaction, serum sickness
Type IV	Delayed-type hypersensitivity	Sensitized T_H1 cells activated to release cytokines upon binding to antigen, resulting in macrophage and cytotoxic T cell accumulation	Contact dermatitis, chronic transplant rejection

Color Plates of Autoimmune Diseases

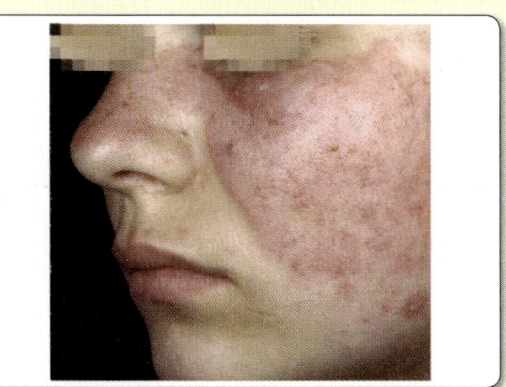

Color plate 1: SLE

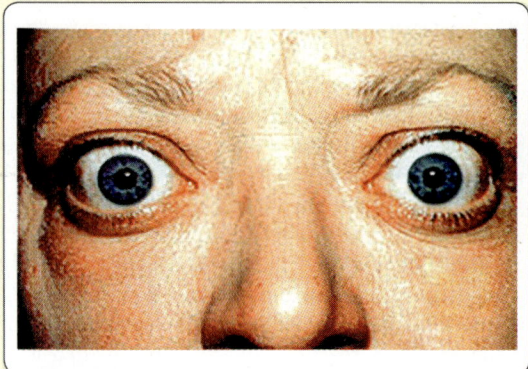

Color plate 2: Graves

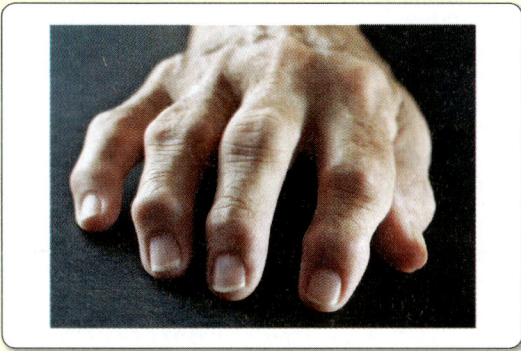

Color plate 3: Arthritis

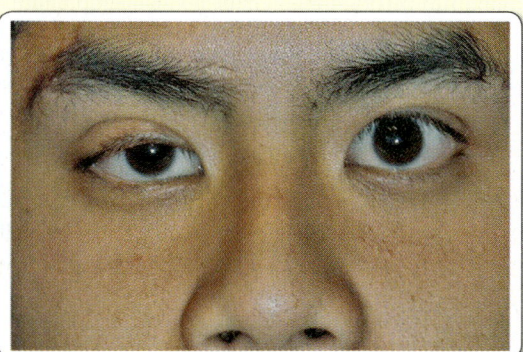

Color plate 4: Myasthenia gravis

Assess Yourself

LONG ANSWER QUESTIONS

1. Define immunity.
2. Explain the types of immunity.

SHORT NOTES

1. Hypersensitivity
2. Types of immunity

MULTIPLE CHOICE QUESTIONS

1. Which antibody crosses placenta?
    - a. IgA
    - b. IgG
    - c. IgE
    - d. IgM

2. Type I hypersensitivity is mediated by which of the following immunoglobulins?
    - a. IgA
    - b. IgG
    - c. IgM
    - d. IgE

3. Zero dose of OPV is given:
    - a. At one month
    - b. At birth
    - c. When child is having diarrhea
    - d. When child is having polio

4. Which of the following is live attenuated vaccine?
    - a. BCG vaccine
    - b. Rabies vaccine
    - c. Diphtheria toxoid
    - d. Tetanus toxoid

5. Which antibody is responsible for allergic responses?
    - a. IgG
    - b. IgA
    - c. IgD
    - d. IgE

6. Anaphylaxis is:
    - a. Type I hypersensitivity
    - b. Type II hypersensitivity
    - c. Type III hypersensitivity
    - d. Type IV hypersensitivity

7. BCG is a:
    - a. Live attenuated vaccine
    - b. Killed vaccine
    - c. Toxoid
    - d. Immunoglobulin

ANSWERS TO MCQS

1. b   **2.** d   **3.** b   **4.** a   **5.** d   **6.** a   **7.** a

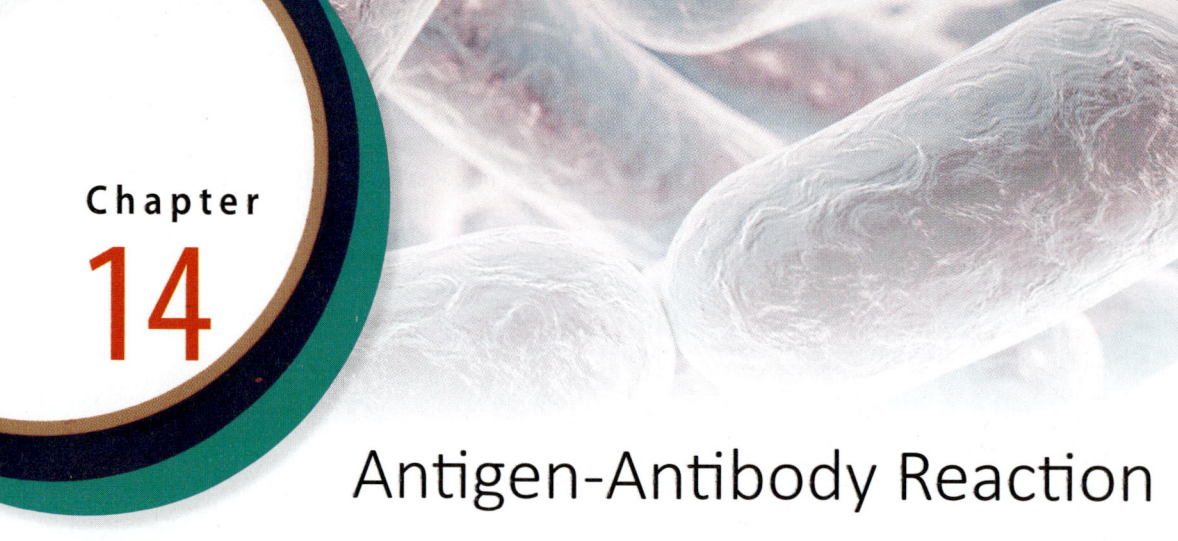

Antigen-Antibody Reaction

INTRODUCTION

Antigens combine with their specific antibodies in a specific and observable manner. The reaction is reversible and complete molecules of antigen and antibody react with each other. While these reactions provide protection to the body against various diseases, they can be used to diagnose infections and detection of antigens or antibodies in the laboratory.

SEROLOGICAL TESTS

Principles of Serological Tests

- Serological diagnosis is usually based on either the demonstration of the presence of specific IgM antibodies or a significant increase in the levels of specific IgG antibodies between two consecutive samples taken 1–4 weeks apart.
- The antigen for the test can be either viable or inactivated virus or some of its components prepared by virological or molecular methods.
- Isotype-specific markers or physical separation are used to demonstrate the isotype of the reacting antibody.

Serological tests based on antigen-antibody reactions are as follows.

PRECIPITATION REACTIONS

When a soluble antigen reacts with an antibody in the presence of electrolytes like sodium chloride (NaCl) at a specific temperature and pH, they form an antigen-antibody complex (in the form of precipitate) that settles down at the bottom of the test tube. This reaction is called precipitation reactions. When this complex does not settles down but remains suspended in the test tube, it is called flocculation.

Ring Test

In this technique, antiserum containing antibodies is put in a narrow test tube and antigen solution is layered over it. A precipitate ring appears where the two liquids meet. It is used for C-reactive protein test and streptococcal grouping.

Flocculation Test

It can be done either on a slide or in a test tube.

- **Slide test:** A drop of inactivated serum of patient is put on a slide and a drop of antigen solution is added over it and they are mixed by shaking. It leads to appearance of suspended complexes called floccules. Venereal Disease Research Laboratory (VDRL) test is an example of slide test and is used to detect antibodies against syphilis.
- **Tube test:** The Kahn test is an example of tube test and was done previously for diagnosis of syphilis.

AGGLUTINATION REACTIONS

In this type of antigen-antibody reaction, a particulate antigen combines with its antibody in the presence of electrolytes like sodium chloride (NaCl) and optimal temperature and pH. There is visible clumping of particles.

Slide Agglutination Test

In this, a drop of antiserum is added to the uniform suspension of antigen and saline on the slide. If immediate clumping is seen, the test is positive. This is generally used for blood group determination and cross matching.

Tube Agglutination Test

In this, the serum is serially diluted by increasing the dilution by two times in a series of test tubes. Particulate antigen is added in equal volume to all the tubes. The highest dilution of serum at which agglutination occurs is the antibody titer. This technique is used in routine in Widal test for diagnosis of typhoid.

COMPLEMENT FIXATION TEST

Complement is absorbed during combinations of antigens and antibodies while taking part in various immunological reactions. This is based on the principle that the antigen-antibody complexes have the ability to 'fix' complement. It is a very sensitive test and can detect even the smallest amounts of antigen and antibody. Diseases like gonorrhea, syphilis, typhus fever, Kala-azar, etc. are diagnosed by this technique.

IMMUNOFLUORESCENCE

Fluorescent dyes absorb invisible ultraviolet light and emit visible green light, which has a longer wavelength. Therefore, if microorganisms or any cell is stained with a fluorescent dye and examined under the microscope with ultraviolet light, they are seen as bright objects against a dark background. This principle is used in fluorescence microscopy. Coons and his colleagues showed that fluorescent dyes can be conjugated to antibodies, leading to their ready detection when attached to an antigen associated with the cell. This method is used for diagnosing rabies virus antigens, syphilis, and detection of autoantibodies.

ENZYME LINKED IMMUNOSORBENT ASSAY (ELISA)

It is an enzyme-based test that can detect either antigens or antibodies in the serum sample of patient. The principle for this method is same as that of immunofluorescence. The only difference is that instead of dyes, enzyme is being used. The enzyme acts on substrate to produce a color in a positive test. This is the most commonly used serological test that is being used to diagnose diseases like tuberculosis, hepatitis B and C, HIV infection, rubella and herpes simplex virus.

USES OF SEROLOGICAL TESTS

For the diagnosis of certain bacterial, parasitic, and viral diseases, including measles, polio, influenza, yellow fever, Rocky mountain spotted fever and infectious mononucleosis.

These are also useful in the detection of autoantibodies (harmful antibodies that attack components of the body) that are involved in autoimmune diseases, such as arthritis.

As a practical mass-screening tool, serological testing has proved valuable in the detection of diseases such syphilis, AIDS and COVID.

Assess Yourself

LONG ANSWER QUESTION

1. Discuss uses of serological tests.

MULTIPLE CHOICE QUESTIONS

1. Ring test is used to detect:
   - a. Streptococcus
   - b. Retrovirus
   - c. Pneumococcus
   - d. Both A and C

2. Kahn test is:
   - a. Slide test
   - b. Ring test
   - c. Tube test
   - d. Complement fixation test

3. Immunofluorescence is used for diagnosing all except:
   - a. Rabies virus
   - b. Syphilis
   - c. Detection of autoantibodies
   - d. Streptococcal infection

4. Complement fixation test is used to diagnose all except:
   - a. Syphilis
   - b. Gonorrhea
   - c. Kala-azar
   - d. Rabies virus

5. Schick test is done for the diagnosis of:
   - a. Rubella
   - b. Measles
   - c. Diphtheria
   - d. Mumps

ANSWERS TO MCQs

1. a **2.** c **3.** d **4.** d **5.** c

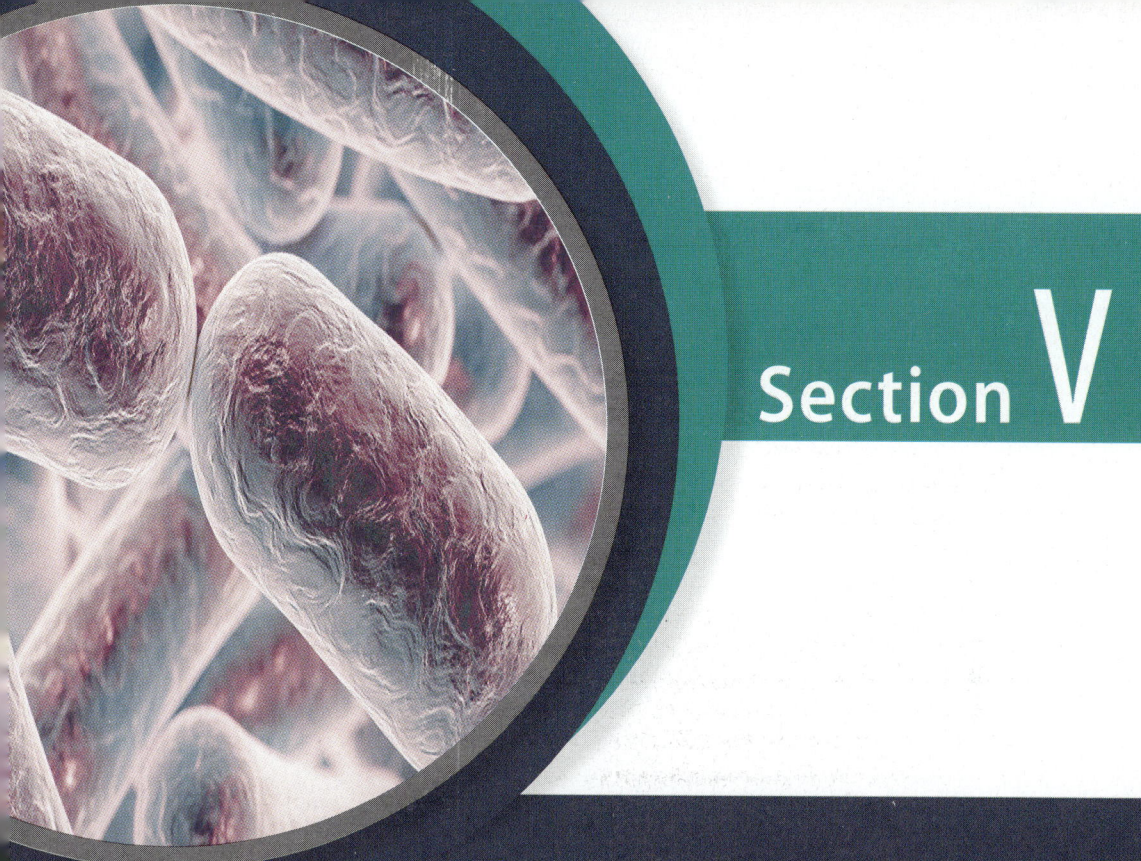

CONTROL OF MICROORGANISMS

Section Summary

Sterilization and Disinfection

INTRODUCTION

Most of the healthcare-associated infections occur because of the hospital premises and the equipment are not properly sterilized and disinfected. Since the microorganisms cause infections, contamination and decay, it is necessary to destroy or limit their population from the required areas. Various microorganisms differ in their susceptibility to physical and chemical agents. The vegetative cells are more susceptible as compared to the bacterial spores towards the effect of physical and chemical agents. There are two processes that are used to remove or destroy microorganisms, disinfection and sterilization. These two methods either reduce the number of bacteria or they completely destroy them.

Terms to Learn

- **Disinfection:** A process that eliminates most or all pathogenic microorganisms from inanimate objects, except bacterial spores.

Contd...

- **Cleaning:** A process that involves removal of visible soil, e.g., organic and inorganic material from objects and surfaces.
- **Decontamination:** A process that involves the removal of pathogenic microorganisms from objects to make them safe to handle or use.
- **Sterilization:** Any process that eliminates, removes, kills, or deactivates all forms of life and other biological agents.

DISINFECTION

Disinfection is the process of eliminating most of the pathogenic microorganisms from inanimate objects. However, it does not cause any effect on the bacterial spores. Many chemical agents are used for this purpose and are known as disinfectants. However, there are many factors that determine the potency of the disinfectants:

- Presence of extraneous material in the area
- Time of action
- Temperature of the medium

- Nature of the microorganisms
- Concentration of the disinfectant
- pH of the medium.

Methods of Disinfection

The most effective methods of disinfection are:

- **Formaldehyde:** Formaldehyde is primarily available as a water-based solution called formalin, which contains 37% formaldehyde by weight and is used as a high-level disinfectant. Formaldehyde acts against bacteria, fungi, viruses and bacterial spores in the aqueous state, as well as in combination with low-temperature steam. It interacts and cross-links with protein, deoxyribonucleic acid (DNA) and ribonucleic acid (RNA) *in vitro*, resulting in the disruption of DNA synthesis. Formaldehyde has been traditionally used to sterilize equipment such as surgical instruments and hemodialyzers in combination with alcohols. Paraformaldehyde, a solid polymer of formaldehyde, is used in combination with low-temperature steam for the disinfection of heat-sensitive medical equipment.
- **Glutaraldehyde:** Glutaraldehyde is a dialdehyde widely used as a potent disinfectant. Its broad spectrum action against bacteria, bacterial spores, fungi and viruses, makes it an ideal chemical for the low-temperature disinfection and sterilization of critical and semi-critical equipment such as endoscopes, dialyzers and surgical tools.
- **Hydrogen peroxide:** Disinfectant solutions containing 7.5% hydrogen peroxide have been widely approved disinfection in healthcare settings. Its broad-spectrum actions against bacteria, viruses, bacterial spores and fungi, combined with its excellent stability and environment-friendly characteristics, have made it the disinfectant of choice for semi-critical and non-critical equipment while being an ideal surface disinfectant.
- **Peracetic acid:** Another emerging alternative to ethylene oxide and aldehyde disinfectants is peracetic acid. Peracetic acid based solutions are considered to be a more potent disinfectant than hydrogen peroxide; are sporicidal, bactericidal, virucidal and fungicidal at low concentrations; and are environment friendly.

- **Hydrogen peroxide/peracetic acid combination:** Peracetic acid, when combined with hydrogen peroxide, was found to be more effective, typically against glutaraldehyde-resistant mycobacteria.
- **Sodium hypochlorite:** Chlorine-releasing agents (CRAs), the most popular sodium hypochlorite solution, are widely used for the disinfection of hard surfaces and blood spillages containing the human immunodeficiency virus (HIV) or hepatitis B virus (HBV). Recently, sodium hypochlorite was designated as the best defense against hospital-acquired and community-acquired *Clostridium difficile* infections.
- **Iodophors:** These are the complexes of iodine and a carrier used as surface disinfectants. Iodophors, such as povidone-iodine, are much more stable, have fewer irritant characteristics and exert effective action against microbes than aqueous iodine solutions.
- **Phenols:** Phenolic disinfectants are effective against bacteria, fungi and viruses but are ineffective against spore-forming bacteria such as *Clostridium difficile*. Phenolic disinfectants act by disrupting the cell membrane of microorganisms.
- **Quaternary ammonium compounds:** These are used for a variety of clinical purposes such as preoperative disinfection, disinfection of non-critical instruments, and hard-surface cleaning and deodorization.

Table 15.1 summarizes the properties of commonly used disinfectants.

STERILIZATION

Sterilization is defined as a process that destroys or eliminates all forms of microbial life like bacteria, spores, fungi and viruses such as hepatitis virus and HIV. Sterilization is done to preserve the substance for a long time without decay. The efficacy of any sterilization process will depend on the nature of the product, the extent and type of any contamination, and the conditions under which the final product has been prepared. Classical sterilization techniques using saturated steam under pressure

TABLE 15.1: Properties of Commonly used Disinfectants

Disinfectant	Activity	Advantages	Disadvantages	Recommendation
Glutaraldehyde	• Broad spectrum microbicidal and sporicidal	• Good compatibility	• Requires activation • Produces irritant fumes	• For fibroscope and respiratory equipment
Orthophthaldehyde	• Broad spectrum microbicidal and sporicidal	• No activation required • No fumes	• Costly • Stains equipment	• For scopes • Alternative to glutaraldehyde
Iodine compounds	• Microbicidal spares • *Mycobacterium tuberculosis* and spores	• Rapid action	• Corrosive to metals, plastic and rubber • Stains items	• As an antiseptic
Alcohols	• Wide microbicidal activity • Nonsporicidal	• Nonstaining	• Flammable	• Hand disinfection • For endoscopes
Phenols	• Wide microbicidal activity • Nonsporicidal	• Easily available • Low cost	• Irritant to skin • Depigmentation	• As surface disinfectant
Quaternary Ammonium compounds	• Microbicidal spares *M. tuberculosis* • Not sporicidal, Not virucidal	• Less irritant • Good detergent property	• Occupational asthma	• As surface disinfectant • For noncritical items
Peracetic acid	Broad spectrum microbicidal and sporicidal	• No activation required • Wide compatibility	• Expansion • Irritant to eye and skin	• For fibroscopes
Chlorines	• Wide microbicidal activity • Nonsporicidal	• Low cost • Fast acting	• Corrosive to metals	• Surface disinfectant to clean blood and body fluid spills
Hydrogen peroxide	• Broad spectrum microbicidal and sporicidal	• No activation required	• Serious eye damage • Incompatible with some metals	• Fogging of operating room • For endoscopes
Formaldehyde	• High level disinfectant	• Noncorrosive	• Pungent odor and irritant fumes • Carcinogenic	• Withdrawn from use

Source: Juwarkar CS. Cleaning and sterilization of anaesthetic equipment. Indian J Anaesth. 2013;57:541-50.

or hot air are the most reliable and should be used whenever possible. Other sterilization methods include filtration, ionizing radiation (gamma and electron-beam radiation), and gas (ethylene oxide, formaldehyde).

Heating in an Autoclave (Steam Sterilization)

Exposure of microorganisms to saturated steam under pressure in an autoclave achieves their

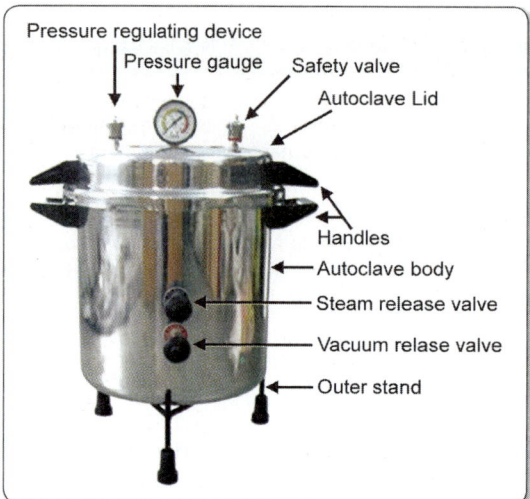

Figure 15.1: Autoclave

destruction by the irreversible denaturation of enzymes and structural proteins. The temperature at which denaturation occurs varies inversely with the amount of water present. Sterilization in saturated steam, thus, requires precise control of time, temperature, and pressure. As displacement of the air by steam is unlikely to be readily achieved, the air should be evacuated from the autoclave before admission of steam. This method should be used whenever possible for aqueous preparations and for surgical dressings and medical devices. The recommendations for sterilization in an autoclave are 15 minutes at 121°–124°C (**Figure 15.1**).

Incineration

This is a safe method of destroying contaminated materials like sputum cups, infected dressings, pathological materials, animal carcasses etc. It is an economical and effective way of destroying materials by complete burning. Polyvinyl chloride (PVC) and polythene can be disposed of in this way except polystyrene materials, which emit dense clouds of smoke and hence, should be autoclaved separately.

Dry-heat Sterilization

In dry-heat processes, the primary lethal process is considered to be oxidation of cell constituents.

Dry-heat sterilization requires a higher temperature than moist heat and a longer exposure time. The method is, therefore, more convenient for heat-stable, non-aqueous materials that cannot be sterilized by steam because of its deleterious effects or failure to penetrate. Such materials include glassware, powders, oils, and some oil-based injectables.

Filtration

Sterilization by filtration is employed mainly for thermolabile solutions. These may be sterilized by passage through sterile bacteria-retaining filters, e.g., membrane filters (cellulose derivatives, etc.), plastic, porous ceramic, or suitable sintered glass filters, or combinations of these. Asbestos-containing filters should not be used.

Exposure to Ionizing Radiation

Sterilization of certain active ingredients, drug products, and medical devices in their final container or package may be achieved by exposure to ionizing radiation in the form of gamma radiation from a suitable radioisotopic source such as ^{60}Co (cobalt 60) or of electrons energized by a suitable electron accelerator. Laws and regulations for protection against radiation must be respected. Gamma radiation and electron beams are used to effect ionization of the molecules in organisms. Mutations are thus formed in the DNA and these reactions alter replication. These processes are very dangerous and only well-trained and experienced staff should decide upon the desirability of their use and should ensure monitoring of the processes.

Gas Sterilization

The active agent of the gas sterilization process can be ethylene oxide or another highly volatile substance. The highly flammable and potentially explosive nature of such agents is a disadvantage unless they are mixed with suitable inert gases to reduce their highly toxic properties and the possibility of toxic residues remaining in treated materials. The whole process is difficult to control and should only be considered if no other sterilization procedure can be used. It must only be carried out under the supervision of highly skilled staff.

Pasteurization

It is a process of making milk and milk products and other food stuffs safe for consumption by destroying all harmful microorganisms like *Mycobacteria*, *Brucella*, diphtheria, *Staphylococcus* and *Salmonella* species. Spores and *Coxiella burnetti* are not destroyed because they are heat resistant.

Different Methods of Pasteurization

- Low-temperature hold method (LTH): Conditions of 63°C for 30 minutes before cooled to 7°C
- High-temperature short-time (HTST): Conditions of 71.5°C for at least 15 seconds before cooled to 10°C
- Ultrahigh-temperature (UHT): 138°C for at least 2 seconds
- Extreme pasteurization
- Kills all microorganisms
- Keeping milk in a closed, sterile container at room temperature

Effect on Foods

- Pasteurization is mild heat treatment. However, minor changes to nutritional and sensorial characteristics are observed. These are as follows:
  - Shelf life of a product increases from a few days or weeks
  - The color of fruit juices deteriorates by enzymic browning (poly phenol oxidase). This browning reaction promoted by the presence of oxygen.
  - Whiteness of raw milk and pasteurized milk differs due to homogenization. Pasteurization has no measurable effects on the color of milk.
  - Pigments in plant and animal products are mostly unaffected.
  - Small loss of volatile aroma compounds during pasteurization of juices.
  - Volatile recovery used to produce high quality juices.
  - The losses of vitamin C and carotene in food are minimized.
  - 5% loss of serum proteins and small changes to vitamin content may be there in milk.

CHEMOTHERAPY AND ANTIBIOTICS

Chemotherapy is the treatment of infectious diseases by administration of drugs or the antibiotics that either kill or inhibit the growth of the causative organisms. The credit of discovery of antibiotics goes to Alexander Fleming, who in 1928, noted that the product of fungi *Penicillium notatum* could inhibit the growth of staphylococci and other organisms. This was purified successfully in 1940 by Florey et al. and was named penicillin. This discovery led to the era of antibiotics and was a major breakthrough in medical history.

The term, Antimicrobial agents, was originally used to denote a chemical substance produced by one microorganism that kills or inhibits the growth of other microbes. The term now applies to both naturally produced substances and those synthesized in the laboratory. Most are produced by either fungi (e.g., penicillin, cephalosporins), Bacillus species (e.g., polymyxin, bacitracin), or Streptomyces species (streptomycin, tetracycline, erythromycin, kanamycin, neomycin, nystatin). Antibiotics are used against bacteria, antifungal agents against fungi, antiviral agents against viruses and so on. Broad-spectrum antibiotics are those that act on both Gram-positive and Gram-negative bacteria.

Action of Antimicrobial Agents

Antimicrobial agents interfere with specific processes that are essential for growth and/or division. They can be separated into groups such as inhibitors of bacterial and fungal cell walls, inhibitors of cytoplasmic membranes, inhibitors of nucleic acid synthesis, and inhibitors of ribosome function. **(Figure 15.2)**

Antimicrobial agents may be either bactericidal, killing the target bacterium or fungus, or bacteriostatic, inhibiting its growth. Bactericidal agents are more effective, but bacteriostatic agents can be extremely beneficial since they permit the normal defenses of the host to destroy the microorganisms.

Mechanism of Action of Antimicrobial Agents

- **Inhibition of cell wall synthesis:** Due to its unique structure and function, the bacterial

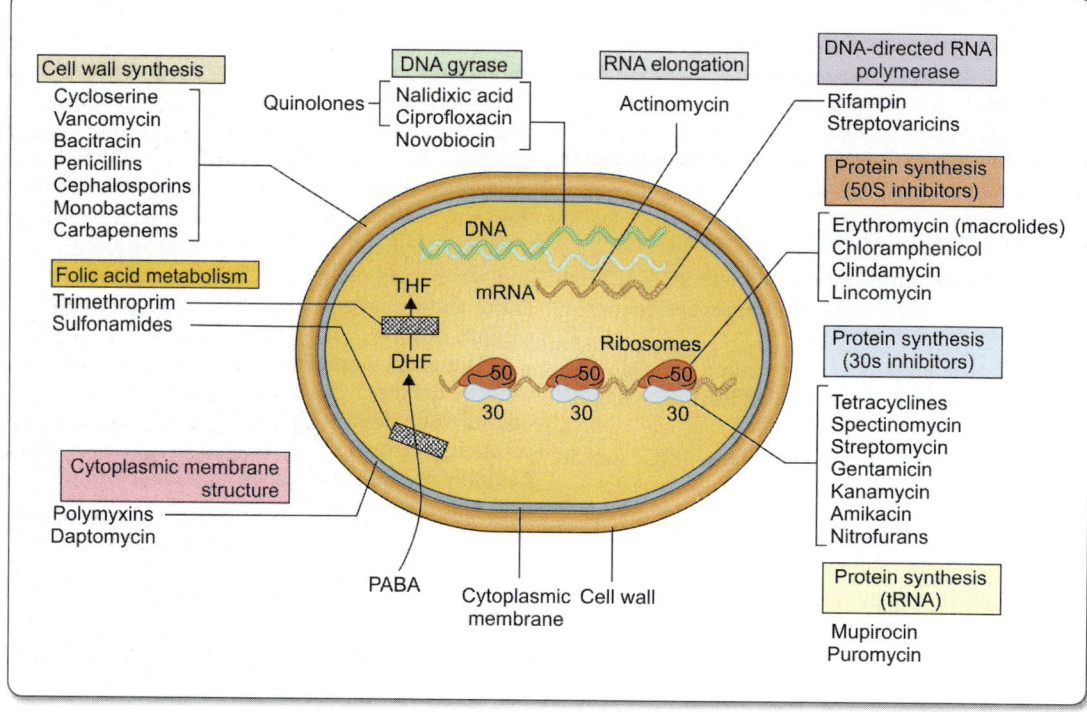

Figure 15.2: Action of antibiotics on bacterial cell

cell wall is an ideal point of attack by selective toxic agents. Some antibiotics, e.g., penicillin, cephalosporins and vancomycin, interfere with cell wall synthesis and cause bacteriolysis.

- **Inhibition of cytoplasmic membrane function:** Some antibiotics cause disruption of the cytoplasm membrane and leakage of cellular proteins and nucleotides leading to cell death. Polymyxins, amphotericin B and nystatin are examples.

- **Inhibition of protein synthesis:** Many antimicrobial chemotherapeutics block protein synthesis by acting on the 30s or 50s subunits of the bacterial ribosome. Examples are chloramphenicol, tetracycline, erythromycin and the aminoglycosides, e.g., tobramycin, gentamycin and streptomycin.

- **Inhibition of nucleic acid synthesis:** These can act on any of the steps of DNA or RNA replication, e.g. quinolones, trimethoprim, rifampicin, nalidixic acid, novobiocin and metronidazole.

- **Competitive inhibition:** The chemotherapeutic agent competes with an essential metabolite for the same enzyme e.g., p-aminobenzoic acid (PABA) is an essential metabolite for many organisms. They use it as a precursor in folic acid synthesis which is essential for nucleic acid synthesis. Sulphonamides are structural analogues to PABA so they enter into the reaction in place of PABA and compete for the active center of the enzyme thus inhibiting folic acid synthesis.

Mode of Action of Common Classes of Antibiotics (Table 15.2)

TABLE 15.2: Classes of Antibiotics and their Properties

Chemical class	Examples	Biological source	Spectrum (effective against)	Mode of action
Beta-lactams (penicillins and cephalosporins)	Penicillin G, Cephalothin	Penicillium notatum and Cephalosporium species	Gram-positive bacteria	Inhibits steps in cell wall (peptidoglycan) synthesis and murein assembly
Semisynthetic penicillin	Ampicillin, Amoxycillin		Gram-positive and Gram-negative bacteria	Inhibits steps in cell wall (peptidoglycan) synthesis and murein assembly
Clavulanic acid	Clavamox is clavulanic acid plus amoxycillin	Streptomyces clavuligerus	Gram-positive and Gram-negative bacteria	"Suicide" inhibitor of beta-lactamases
Monobactams	Aztreonam	Chromobacter violaceum	Gram-positive and Gram-negative bacteria	Inhibits steps in cell wall (peptidoglycan) synthesis and murein assembly
Carboxypenems	Imipenem	Streptomyces cattleya	Gram-positive and Gram-negative bacteria	Inhibits steps in cell wall (peptidoglycan) synthesis and murein assembly
Aminoglycosides	Streptomycin	Streptomyces griseus	Gram-positive and Gram-negative bacteria	Inhibit translation (protein synthesis)
	Gentamicin	Micromonospora species	Gram-positive and Gram-negative bacteria esp. Pseudomonas	Inhibit translation (protein synthesis)
Glycopeptides	Vancomycin	Streptomyces orientales	Gram-positive bacteria, esp. Staphylococcus aureus	Inhibits steps in murein (peptidoglycan) biosynthesis and assembly

PREVENTING CROSS INFECTION IN HOSPITALS MEDICAL AND SURGICAL ASEPSIS

Asepsis is defined as freedom from infection or infectious material or the absence of viable pathogenic organisms. It can be broadly divided into Medical asepsis and Surgical asepsis. Medical asepsis is the reduction of the number of disease-causing agents and their spread. The complete elimination of the disease-causing agents and their spores from the surface of an object is called the surgical asepsis. Both methods are helpful to prevent cross infections in hospitals.

Medical Asepsis

Medical asepsis is also called as clean technique. It is aimed at destroying pathological organisms after they leave the body and is employed in the care of patients with infectious diseases to prevent reinfection of the patient and to avoid the spread of infection from one person to another. Hand hygiene, skin preparation prior to the injection of a subcutaneous medication, and the administration of all medications except those given intravenously, are examples of the application of medical asepsis principles into nursing care practices. It is achieved by the following practices:

- Isolation of the patient
- Hand washing
- Administering preventive vaccination
- Increasing the awareness among visitors and relatives
- Using the protective equipment like gloves, masks and gowns
- Using chemical agents for disinfection

Surgical Asepsis

The complete elimination of the disease-causing agents and their spores from the surface of an object is called surgical asepsis. Surgical asepsis is used for wound care, during all invasive procedures including surgical procedures and other invasive procedures such as endoscopy, for the administration of intravenous medications, for wound care, and for the insertion of an indwelling urinary catheter as well as other internally placed tubes like central lines and peripheral intravenous lines.

Measures that are taken to perform surgical asepsis include sterilization of all instruments, drapes, and all other inanimate objects that may come in contact with the surgical wound.

Thus, both play an important role in maintaining suitable environment needed for patient care.

? Assess Yourself

LONG ANSWER QUESTIONS

1. What are methods of sterilization?
2. Discuss the types of sterilization.
3. Explain autoclaving method of sterilization.
4. Explain the different methods of sterilization.
5. Define sterilization. Explain the physical methods of sterilization.
6. How will you prevent cross infection in hospital?

SHORT NOTES

1. Ionizing radiation
2. Pasteurization
3. Disinfection
4. Steam sterilization

MULTIPLE CHOICE QUESTIONS

1. Which of the following is moist heat method of sterilization?
   a. Autoclave
   b. Hot air oven
   c. Ultraviolet radiation
   d. Incineration
2. The method of killing of all microorganisms including their spores is known as:
   a. Sterilization
   b. Disinfection
   c. Incineration
   d. Lysis

Contd...

Assess Yourself

3. The method of reducing the number of pathogens from any article, surface or medium is called as:
   a. Sterilization
   b. Disinfection
   c. Incineration
   d. Lysis

4. Which of the following is moist heat method of sterilization?
   a. Boiling
   b. Autoclaving
   c. Hot air oven
   d. Both a & b

5. Alcohols, aldehydes, phenols, etc. are:
   a. Chemical methods of sterilization
   b. Physical methods of sterilization
   c. Dry heat method of sterilization
   d. Moist heat method of sterilization

6. Hot air oven is used for sterilizing _____materials.
   a. Glassware (like petri dishes, flasks, pipettes, and test tubes)
   b. Powders (like starch, zinc oxide, and sulfadiazine)
   c. Materials that contain oils. Metal equipment (like scalpels, scissors, and blades)
   d. All of the above

7. Culture media is sterilized by which of the following method?
   a. Autoclaving
   b. Hot air oven
   c. Boiling
   d. Ionizing radiation

ANSWERS TO MCQS

1. a   **2.** a   **3.** b   **4.** d   **5.** a   **6.** d   **7.** a

Section V • Control of Microorganisms

Chapter

16

Biomedical Waste Management

INTRODUCTION

All human activities produce waste. We all know that such waste may be dangerous and needs safe disposal. Industrial waste, sewage and agricultural waste pollute water, soil and air. It can also be dangerous to human beings and environment. Similarly, hospitals and other health care facilities generate lots of waste which can transmit infections, particularly HIV, Hepatitis B and C and Tetanus, to the people who handle it or come in contact with it.

BIOMEDICAL WASTE

Biomedical waste means "any solid and/or liquid waste including its container and any intermediate product, which is generated during the diagnosis, treatment or immunization of human beings or animals". Biomedical waste poses hazard due to two principal reasons—the first is infectivity and the other, toxicity.

Biomedical waste consists of:
- Human anatomical waste like tissues, organs and body parts

- Animal wastes generated during research from veterinary hospitals
- Microbiology and biotechnology wastes
- Waste sharp instruments like hypodermic needles, syringes, scalpels and broken glass
- Discarded medicines and cytotoxic drugs
- Soiled waste such as dressing, bandages, plaster casts, material contaminated with blood, tubes and catheters
- Liquid waste from any of the infected areas
- Incineration ash and other chemical wastes

Different Types of Biomedical Wastes According to WHO

The World Health Organisation (WHO) has classified medical wastes according to their weight, density and constituents into different categories. These are:
- **Infectious:** Material-containing pathogens in sufficient concentrations or quantities that, if exposed, can cause diseases. This includes waste from surgery and autopsies on patients with infectious diseases, sharps, disposable needles, syringes, saws, blades, broken glasses, nails or any other item that could cause a cut.

- **Pathological:** Tissues, organs, body parts, human flesh, fetuses, blood and body fluids, drugs and chemicals that are returned from wards, spilled, outdated, contaminated, or are no longer required
- **Radioactive:** Solids, liquids and gaseous waste contaminated with radioactive substances used in diagnosis and treatment of diseases like toxic goiter
- **Others:** Waste from the offices, kitchens, rooms, including bed linen, utensils, paper, etc.

BIOMEDICAL WASTE MANAGEMENT

The biomedical waste management requires its categorization as a first step. The biomedical waste rules classify the biomedical waste into 9 categories. **(Table 16.1)**

The key to minimization and effective management of biomedical waste is segregation (separation) and identification of the waste. The most appropriate way of identifying the categories of biomedical waste is by sorting the waste into color-coded plastic bags or containers. Biomedical waste should be segregated into containers/bags at the point of generation **(Figure 16.1 and Table 16.1)**.

Collection of Biomedical Waste

Collection of biomedical waste should be done as per biomedical waste (management and handling) rules. At ordinary room temperature, the collected waste should not be stored for >24 hours.

Transportation

Within hospital, waste routes must be designated to avoid the passage of waste through patient care areas. Separate time should be marked for transportation of biomedical waste to reduce chances of its mixing with general waste. Desiccated wheeled containers, trolleys or carts should be used to transport the waste/plastic bags to the site of storage/treatment.

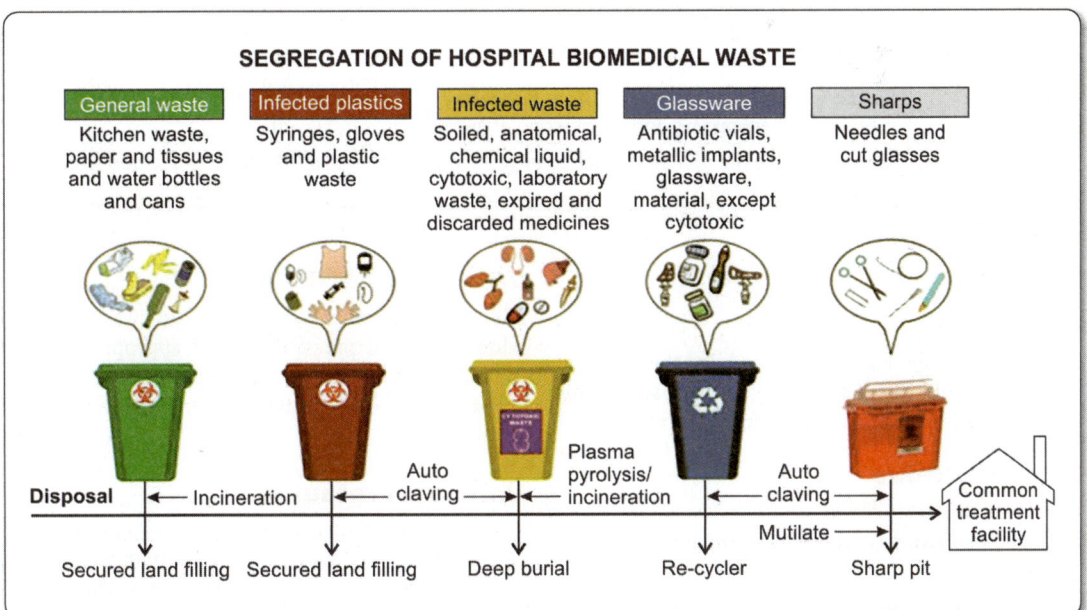

Figure 16.1: Segregation of biomedical waste

TABLE 16.1: Categories of Biomedical Waste Schedule – I

Category	Description of waste category	Treatment and disposal
Category 1	**Human anatomical waste:** Human tissues, organs, body parts.	Incineration/deep burial
Category 2	**Animal waste:** Animal tissues, organs, body parts, carcasses, bleeding parts, fluid, blood and experimental animals used in research, waste generated by veterinary hospitals colleges, discharge from hospitals, animal houses.	Incineration/deep burial
Category 3	**Microbiology and biotechnology waste:** Wastes from laboratory cultures, stocks of specimens of live microorganism live or attenuated vaccines, human and animals cell culture used in research, infectious agents from research and industrial laboratories, wastes from production of biological, toxins, dishes and devices used for transfer of cultures.	Autoclaving/microwaving/incineration
Category 4	**Waste sharps:** Needles, syringes, scalpels, blades, glass, etc. that may cause puncture and cuts. This includes both used and unused sharps.	Disinfecting (chemical treatment/autoclaving/microwaving and mutilation/shredding)
Category 5	**Discarded medicine and cytotoxic drugs:** Wastes comprising of outdated, contaminated and discarded medicines.	Incineration/destruction and drugs disposal in secured landfills
Category 6	**Soiled waste:** Items contaminated with bloods fluids including cotton, dressings, soiled plaster casts, linens, bedding, other materials contaminated with blood.	Incineration/autoclaving/microwaving
Category 7	**Solid waste:** Waste generated from disposable items other than the waste sharps such as tubing, catheters, intravenous sets, etc.	Disinfecting/autoclaving/microwaving and mutilation/shredding
Category 8	**Liquid waste:** Waste generated from laboratory and washing, cleaning, housekeeping and disinfecting activities.	Disinfecting/discharge into drains
Category 9	**Incineration ash:** Ash from incineration of any biomedical waste.	Disposal of secured landfill

Treatment of Hospital Waste

General Waste

The 85% of the waste generated in the hospital belongs to this category. The safe disposal of this waste is the responsibility of the local authority.

Biomedical Waste

- Deep burial
- Autoclave and microwave treatment
- Shredding
- Secured landfill
- Incineration

SAFETY MEASURES

All the generators of biomedical waste should adopt universal precautions and appropriate safety measures while doing therapeutic and diagnostic activities and also while handling the biomedical waste.

Universal Precautions

- Assume that all patients/specimens are potentially infective for human immunodeficiency virus (HIV)/hepatitis B virus (HBV) and other blood-borne pathogens.

- All blood specimens and body fluids stored should be placed in a leak-proof impervious bag for transportation to the laboratory.
- Use gloves while handling blood, body fluid specimens and other objects disposed to them. If there is likelihood of spattering, use face masks, gloves and goggles.
- Wear laboratory coat or gown while working in the laboratory. Wrap-around gowns should be preferred. These should not be taken outside the laboratory.
- Never try to pipette by mouth. Mechanical pipetting devices should be used.
- Decontaminate the laboratory work surfaces with an appropriate disinfectant after spillage of blood or other body fluids and when the procedures are completed.
- Limit use of needles and syringes to situations for which there are no alternatives.
- All the potentially contaminated material of the laboratory should be decontaminated before disposal or reprocessing.

- Always wash hands after completing work and remove all protective clothing before leaving the laboratory.

Personal Protection

- Immunization against hepatitis B and tetanus shall be given to all hospital staff.
- All the generators of Biomedical waste should adopt universal precautions and appropriate safety measures while doing therapeutic and diagnostic activities and also while handling the biomedical waste.
- All the sanitation workers engaged in the handling and transporting should be made aware of the risks involved in handling the biomedical waste.
- Any worker reporting with an accident/injury due to handling of biomedical waste should be given prompt first aid. Necessary investigations and follow up action as per requirement may be carried out.

Section V • Control of Microorganisms

Assess Yourself

LONG ANSWER QUESTION

1. What do you mean by biomedical waste and how do you segregate it?

MULTIPLE CHOICE QUESTIONS

1. Discarded medicine comes in which category of biomedical waste:
   - a. Category 1
   - b. Category 3
   - c. Category 5
   - d. Category 7

2. Human anatomical waste should be treated by:
   - a. Incineration
   - b. Autoclaving
   - c. Microwaving
   - d. Shredding

3. Yellow plastic bag contains wastes of all the categories below except:
   - a. Category 6
   - b. Category 7
   - c. Category 1
   - d. Category 3

4. Red plastic bags should be treated by the following except:
   - a. Incineration
   - b. Autoclaving
   - c. Chemical treatment
   - d. Microwaving

5. Which immunization is necessary for hospital staff?
   - a. DPT
   - b. Hepatitis C
   - c. Hepatitis A
   - d. Hepatitis B

ANSWERS TO MCQs

1. c **2.** a **3.** b **4.** a **5.** d

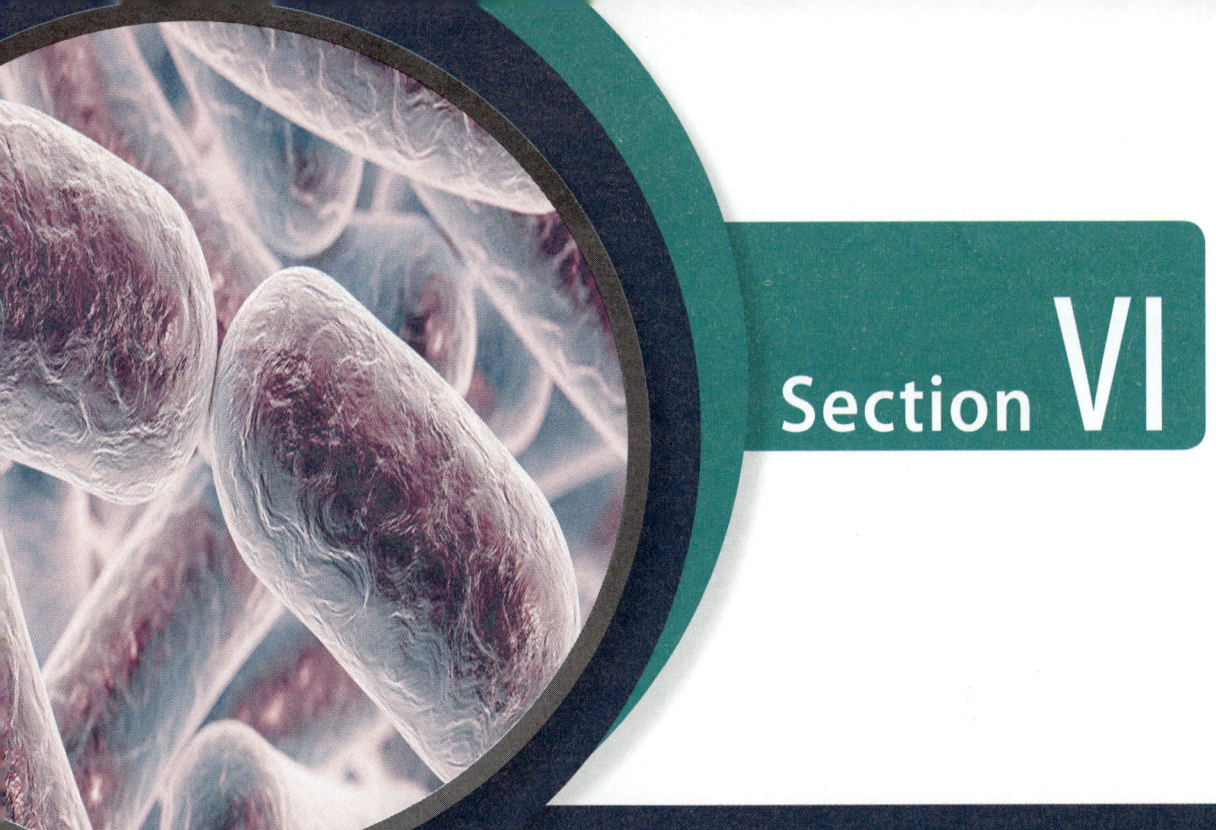

Section VI

PRACTICAL MICROBIOLOGY

Section Summary

Microscope

INTRODUCTION

Most of the microorganisms are invisible to naked eye. Hence, it qualifies for the requirement of a device that can magnify them and help us study their morphology to understand them. Microscope is the device that was invented for this purpose.

PARTS OF A MICROSCOPE

Although a magnifying glass technically qualifies as a simple light microscope, today's high-power—or compound—microscopes use two sets of lenses to give users a much higher level of magnification, along with greater clarity. The first set of lenses are the oculars, or eyepieces, that the viewer looks into; the second set of lenses are the objectives, the lenses closest to the object (specimen). Before using a microscope, it is important to know the functions of each part **(Figure 17.1)**.

- **Eyepieces:** The eyepieces are the lenses at the top that the viewer looks through; they are usually 10X or 15X. To get the total magnification level, multiply the magnification of the objective used (ex: 10X eyepiece × 40X objective = 400X total magnification).
- **Tube:** Where the eyepieces are dropped in. Also, they connect the eyepieces to the objective lenses.

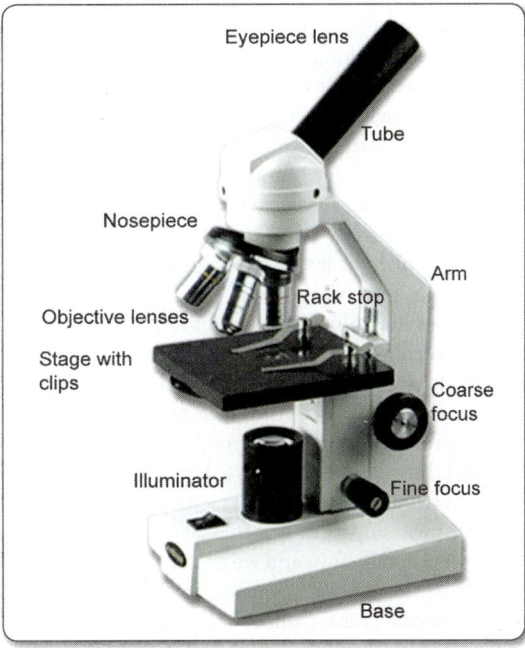

Figure 17.1: Parts of a microscope

- **Base:** The bottom of the microscope on which the microscope stands on.
- **Arm:** Structural element that connects the head of the microscope to the base.

- **Stage:** The flat platform that supports the slides. Stage clips hold the slides in place. If the microscope has a mechanical stage, the slide is controlled by turning two knobs instead of having to move it manually. One knob moves the slide left and right, the other moves it forward and backward.

- **Illuminator:** A steady light source that shines up through the slide. Mirrors are sometimes used in lieu of a built-in light. If the microscope has a mirror, it is used to reflect light from an external light source up through the bottom of the stage.

- **Nose piece:** This circular structure is where the different objective lenses are screwed in. To change the magnification power, simply rotate the turret.

- **Objective lenses:** Usually there are three or four objective lenses on a microscope. The most common ones are 4X (shortest lens), 10X, 40X and 100X (longest lens). The higher power objectives (starting from 40x) are spring loaded. Spring loaded objective lenses will retract if the objective lens hits a slide, preventing damage to both the lens and the slide. All quality microscopes have achromatic, parcentered, parfocal lenses. In addition, to get the greatest clarity at high levels of magnification, one will need a microscope with an Abbe condenser. Lenses are color coded and are interchangeable between microscopes.

- **Rack stop:** This feature determines how far up the stage can go. Setting the rack stop is useful in preventing the slide from coming too far up and hitting the objective lens. Normally, this adjustment is set at the factory, and changing the rack stop is only necessary if the slides are exceptionally thin and we are unable to focus the specimen at higher powers.

- **Condenser lens:** Condenser lenses focus the light that shines up through the slide, and are useful for attaining sharp images at magnifications of 400X and above. If the maximum power of the microscope is 400X, a stage mounted 0.65 numerical aperture (NA) condenser is ideal, since it gives greater clarity without having to be focused separately. However, if the microscope goes to 1000X or above, focusable condenser lens with an NA of 1.25 or greater is needed. Most microscopes that go up to 1000X come equipped with an Abbe condenser, which can be focused by moving it up and down. The Abbe condenser should be set closest to the slide at 1000X, and moved further away as the magnification level gets lower.

- **Diaphragm or iris:** The diaphragm or iris is located under the stage and is an apparatus that can be adjusted to vary the intensity and size, of the cone of light that is projected through the slide. As there is no set rule on which setting to use for a particular power, the setting depends on the transparency of the specimen and the degree of contrast one desires in the image.

HANDLING AND CARE OF MICROSCOPE

- Hold a microscope firmly by the stand, only.
- While picking the microscope and transporting it to one place to another, grab the arm with one hand and place your other hand on the bottom of the base.
- Always make sure the stage and lenses are clean before putting the microscope away.
- Never touch the lenses with fingers. Use lens paper to clean the glass.
- Focus smoothly; don't try to speed through the focusing process or force anything.
- Lower the stage before removing a slide.
- Turn off the power at the end of the day, and unplug the microscope to protect it from a power surge.
- Do not leave lens ports uncovered; use the port cover or sealing tape.
- After finishing the work, rotate the nosepiece so that it's on the low power objective, roll the nosepiece so that it's all the way down to the stage.
- Cover the microscope well to avoid dust contamination.
- Clean all slides, materials, and work area after finishing the work.
- The microscope must be stored in dry conditions when not in use to prevent fungal growth on glass surfaces.

USES OF MICROSCOPE

- Microscopes have helped humankind in the medical field as they facilitate viewing the various microorganisms like viruses, bacteria and deadly microorganisms. Studying their structure helps in identifying their cures as well.
- Forensics also use microscopes to collect and study evidence from crime scenes.
- It helps in tissue analysis. If a section of tissue is taken for analysis, histologists can use a microscope in combination with other tools to determine if the sample is cancerous.

- Field biologists monitor the health of a particular ecosystem, such as a stream, by using microscopes to identify the number and diversity of organisms in a particular region over time.
- Research scientists find microscopes an invaluable tool when they study the function of proteins within cells.
- Powerful microscopes such as atomic force microscopes have aided scientists in studying the surfaces of individual atoms.

Assess Yourself

SHORT NOTE

1. Microscope

MULTIPLE CHOICE QUESTIONS

1. The magnification level is found by:
   a. Dividing the magnification of objective by eyepiece
   b. Multiplying the magnification of objective and eyepiece
   c. Adding the magnification of both objective and eyepiece
   d. Subtracting the magnification of eyepiece from the objective

2. Nose piece is:
   a. A circular structure
   b. A rectangular structure
   c. A rhomboid structure
   d. None

3. Condenser lens are used for attaining the magnification above:
   a. 200X
   b. 600X
   c. 100X
   d. 400X

4. Diaphragm is located:
   a. Above the stage
   b. Under the stage
   c. near the nose piece
   d. Near the objective

5. Electron microscope was discovered by:
   a. Ruska
   b. Joseph Lister
   c. Louis
   d. Pasteur

ANSWERS TO MCQS

1. b   2. a   3. d   4. b   5. a

Staining and Examination of Slides

INTRODUCTION

As bacteria are not visible to naked eyes, staining becomes an important method for examination. Smear made from bacterial cultures or specimens is first air dried and then heat fixed by flaming the slide from underneath. Heat kills and fixes the bacteria on the slide. Various techniques are employed for the same that are discussed below.

STAINING TECHNIQUES

Smear Preparation

- On a glass slide, the culture is mixed in a drop of normal saline and spread thinly.
- It is allowed to air dry and then fixed by heat of Bunsen burner.
- The heat fixing kills, hardens and fixes the bacteria to surface of slide.
- It is due to the coagulation of bacterial protein.
- The overheating of smear is to be avoided as it will distort the morphology of cells.

Fixed, stained preparations are most frequently used for the observation of the morphological characteristics of bacteria.

Advantages

The advantages of this method are:
- The cells are made clearly visible after they are properly stained with suitable dyes.
- Differences between cells of different species and within same species can be demonstrated by using appropriate differential staining solutions.

SIMPLE STAINING

Dyes like methylene blue or basic fuchsin provide color contrast when mixed with bacterial samples, although same color is acquired by all types of bacteria.

Negative Staining

Bacteria are mixed with dyes like India ink or nigrosine that provides a uniformly colored background against, which unstained bacteria are clearly visible. This technique is mainly used to demonstrate capsules. It is also used to see cell size and arrangement of cells.

DIFFERENTIAL STAINING

When different colors are used in staining of a specimen, they give different colors to bacterial components and different bacteria. This method is used widely. Two differential staining techniques used most often are: Gram's staining and acid-fast staining.

Gram Staining

This method of differential staining differentiates the bacteria into two large groups. The one group is called as Gram positive organisms and they retain primary dye, i.e. crystal violet. Another group is called as Gram negative organisms and they take up the counterstain, i.e. safranin.

Principle

In 1884, Christian Gram introduced this test and Hucker modified it in 1921. The basic principle of Gram staining is based on the difference in the cell wall composition of different bacteria. Certain bacteria retain crystal violet color in their cell wall due to high peptidoglycan content whereas some bacteria do not retain it due to low lipid content and take safranin as counterstain. The one that takes primary stain appear purple in color and are Gram-positive and others, which takes counterstain, are Gram-negative organisms.

Mechanism

The Gram-positive cells retain the basic dye more strongly than Gram-negative bacteria. The protoplasm of the cell turns more acidic when iodine is applied on the smear and it fixes the dye in the cell. Explanation for the Gram reaction is that the cell wall of Gram-negative is thinner than the Gram-positive bacteria. Experimental evidences also suggest that the Gram negative cell wall porosity is increased, which permits the decolorizer to remove the crystal violet and iodine complex. Later on, these bacteria take up the counter stain. The cell walls of Gram-positive bacteria have lower lipid content and get dehydrated when treated with alcohol. The pore size decreases and permeability is reduced, which does not permit crystal violet to leave the cell wall of Gram-positive bacteria. Therefore, these bacteria retain the purple color of crystal violet.

Procedure

Smear Preparation

It is prepared by taking a drop of normal saline on a clean slide. A colony from the solid media plate is picked with the help of inoculating wire loop and is emulsified in normal saline. Now after air drying, the smear is heat fixed and is then subjected to staining procedure.

Staining

- Flood the fixed smear with the crystal violet solution and leave it for one minute.
- After pouring out crystal violet, rinse in running water gently so that the dye is not washed off totally.
- Pour iodine solution on the smear and leave it for one minute.
- Rinse gently in water.
- Decolorization is done with alcohol by keeping it on the smear for 30 seconds.
- Again rinse with flowing water.
- Safranin is used as counterstain and is kept on the smear for 30 seconds.
- Again rinse the slide in running water after removing excess of counterstain.
- Air dry the slide and examine under the oil immersion objective of a microscope.

Interpretation of Results

The Gram-positive organisms look purple in color and Gram-negative are pink.

Acid-fast Staining

This is another method for differentiating acid-fast from non-acid-fast bacteria. The method was introduced by Paul Ehrlich in 1882 but modified by Ziehl Neelsen. It is also known as Ziehl Neelsen staining method. The method is very useful in staining *Mycobacterium tuberculosis* and *Mycobacterium leprae*. These bacteria do not take the simple stains due to the presence of variety of fatty acids, i.e., mycolic acid in their cell wall. But when stained with hot concentrated carbol fuchsin the organisms stain bright red.

Method

- Prepare a smear from the purulent portion of the specimen on a glass slide. The specimen should be a morning sample.
- Air dry it, followed by heat fixation.
- Pour carbol fuchsin on the smear so that it covers the smear thoroughly.
- Now heat it gently till steam rises and continue it for 5 minutes without burning the smear.
- Let it cool down and wash it with running water.
- Decolorize with acid alcohol solution, i.e. 3% HCl in alcohol or 20–25% of sulphuric acid in water (v/v) for 3 minutes.
- Wash in running water and drain. Repeat decolorization until smear is light pink in color.
- Pour methylene blue as counter stain for 2 minutes.
- Then drain off the stain and wash again with water. Let it dry and observe under oil immersion objective with a drop of oil on the smear.

Interpretation of Result

The acid-fast tubercle bacilli appear as bright red rods with a blue background.

EXAMINATION OF SMEARS

- Place a drop of blood, about 2–3 mm in diameter approximately 1 cm from one end of slide.
- Place the slide on a flat surface, and hold the other end between your left thumb and forefinger.

- With your right hand, place the smooth clean edge of a second (spreader) slide on the specimen slide, just in front of the blood drop.
- Hold the spreader slide at a 30°–45° angle, and draw it back against the drop of blood
- Allow the blood to spread almost to the edges of the slide.
- Push the spread forward with one light, smooth moderate speed. A thin film of blood in the shape of tongue **(Figure 18.1)**.
- Label one edge with patient name, lab id and date.
- The slides should be rapidly air dried by waving the slides or using an electrical fan.

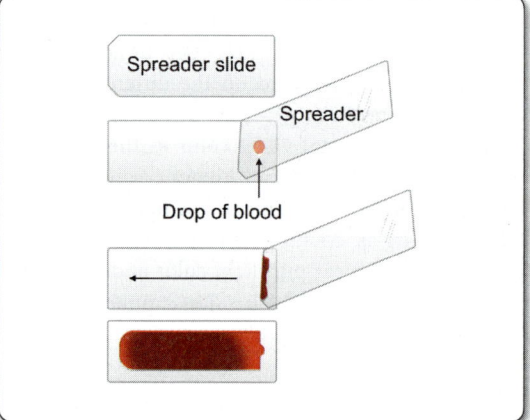

Figure 18.1: Preparation of smears

Assess Yourself

LONG ANSWER QUESTIONS

1. How will you prepare and examine smear?
2. What is acid-fast staining? Write a note on it.
3. Write a note on Gram staining.

MULTIPLE CHOICE QUESTIONS

1. The most common staining technique used to distinguish between Gram +ve and Gram−ve bacteria is:
   a. Gram staining
   b. Ziehl-Neelsen staining
   c. Acid-fast staining
   d. None of the above

2. The most common staining technique used to stain Mycobacteria species is:
   a. Gram staining
   b. Ziehl-Neelsen staining
   c. Acid-fast staining
   d. None of the above

3. The microorganism that can be acid-fast stained is:
   a. Tubercle bacilli
   b. Lepra bacilli
   c. Nocardia
   d. All of the above

4. Substance used for decolorizing gram stain is:
   a. Acetone
   b. Formaldehyde
   c. Gluteraldehyde
   d. Cidex

5. Stain used in acid-fast staining is:
   a. Dilute carbol fuchsin
   b. Concentrated carbol fuchsin
   c. Methyl violet
   d. Iodine

ANSWERS TO MCQs

1. a   2. b   3. d   4. a   5. b

INDEX

Refer 'f' for figure and 't' for table, respectively.

R

S

Nursing Knowledge Tree

An Initiative by CBS Nursing Division

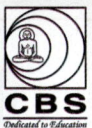

CBS
Dedicated to Education

Nursing Catalogue 2021

Update: February, 2021

Books for All

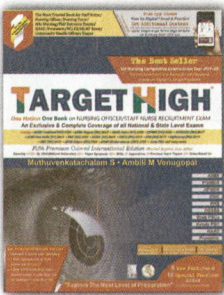

ISBN: 978-93-89261-98-1
Pages: 1350   5/e, 2020-21
MRP: ₹1350/-

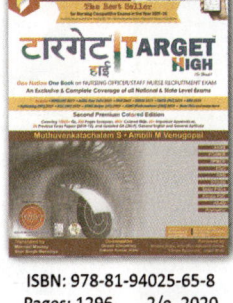

ISBN: 978-81-94025-65-8
Pages: 1296   2/e, 2020
MRP: ₹1199/-

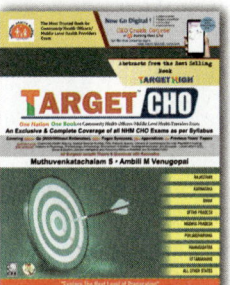

ISBN: 978-81-940256-0-3
Pages: 470   1/e, 2020
MRP: ₹495/-

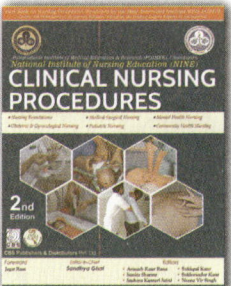

ISBN: 978-93-89261-97-4
Pages: 1296   2/e, 2019
MRP: ₹1295/-

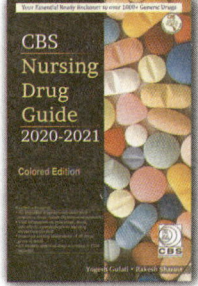

ISBN: 978-93-88178-53-2
Pages: 1670   1/e, 2020
MRP: ₹1050/-

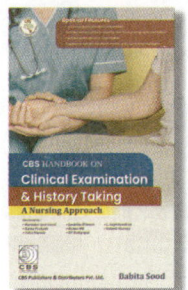

ISBN: 978-81-948693-9-9
Pages: 408   1/e, 2021
MRP: ₹350/-

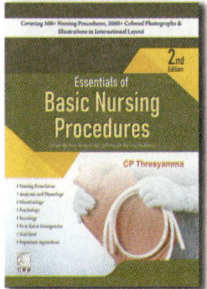

ISBN: 978-81-94523-47-5
Pages: 1016   2/e, 2020
MRP: ₹795/

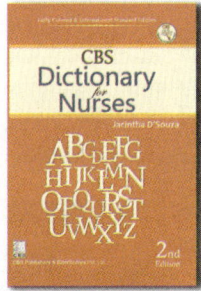

ISBN: 978-81-23927-16-9
Pages: 872   2/e, 2017
MRP: ₹375/-

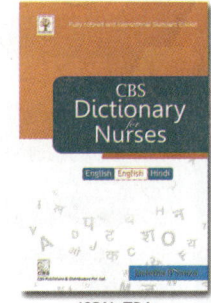

ISBN: TBA
Pages: 1100 (T)   1/e, 2021
MRP: TBA

Read, Review & Buy

Now, buying CBS Nursing Books is extra convenient with 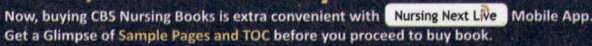 Mobile App.
Get a Glimpse of Sample Pages and TOC before you proceed to buy book.

Download the App from Google Playstore or scan here to download

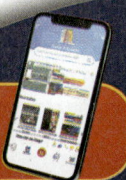

Community Health Nursing

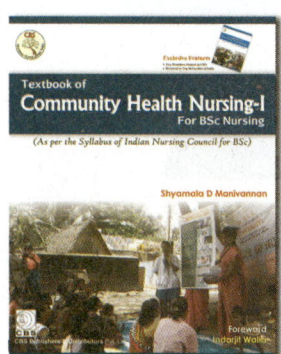

ISBN: 978-81-23927-01-5
Pages: 508   1/e, 2018
MRP: ₹750/-

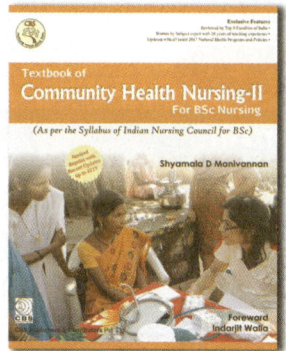

ISBN: 978-93-86827-22-7
Pages: 326   1/e, 2018
MRP: ₹450/-

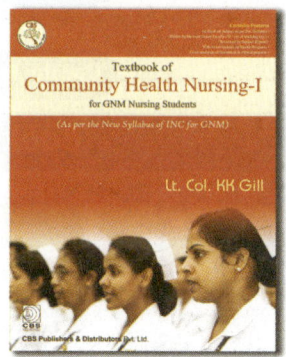

ISBN: 978-93-86827-17-3
Pages: 544   1/e, 2018
MRP: ₹550/-

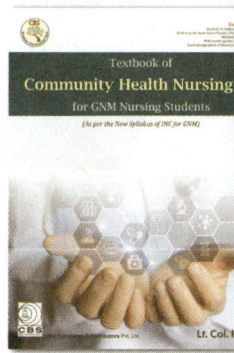

ISBN: 978-93-88178-57
Pages: 480   1/e, 2
MRP: ₹525/-

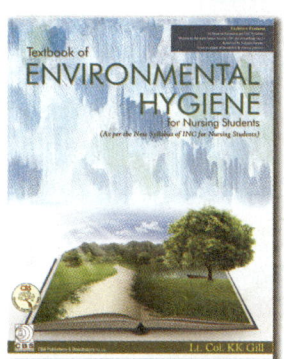

ISBN: 978-93-88178-56-3
Pages: 110   1/e, 2018-19
MRP: ₹225/-

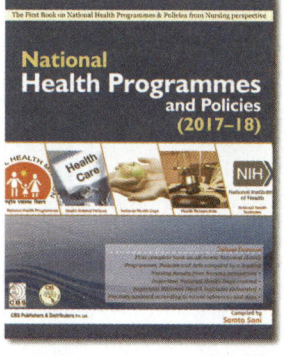

ISBN: 978-93-86310-43-9
Pages: 584   1/e, 2018
MRP: ₹675/-

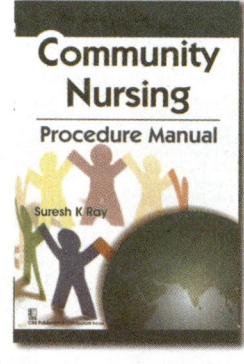

ISBN: 978-81-23929-35-4
Pages: 179   1/e, 2017
MRP: ₹265/-

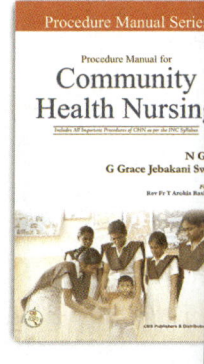

ISBN: 978-81-948693
Pages: 136   1/e, 2
MRP: TBA

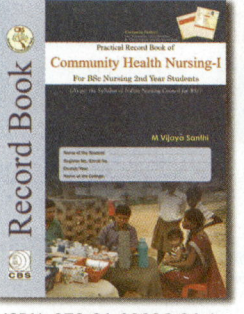

ISBN: 978-81-23926-84-1
Pages: 388   1/e, 2016
MRP: ₹450/-

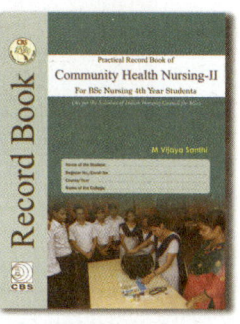

ISBN: 978-93-88108-77-5
Pages: 544   1/e, 2018-19
MRP: ₹575/-

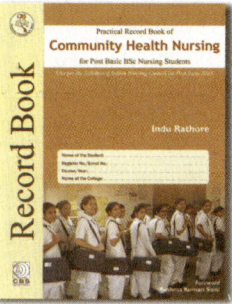

ISBN: 978-93-86827-06-7
Pages: 390   1/e, 2017
MRP: ₹475/-

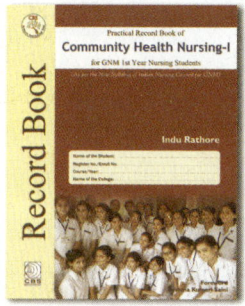

ISBN: 978-93-86827-07-4
Pages: 252   1/e, 2020
MRP: ₹350/-

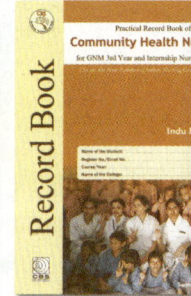

ISBN: 978-93-86827-
Pages: 320   1/e, 201
MRP: ₹395/-

 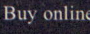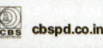 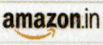 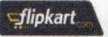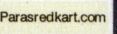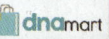

Nursing Foundation

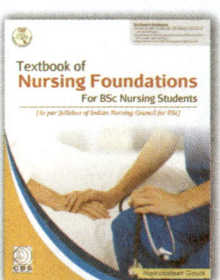
ISBN: 978-93-88108-94-2
Pages: 700   1/e, 2020
MRP: ₹950/-

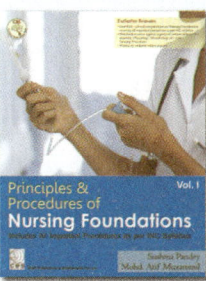
ISBN: 978-93-88108-95-9
Pages: 392   1/e, 2018
MRP: ₹625/-

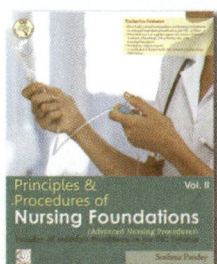
ISBN: 978-93-89261-87-5
Pages: 272   1/e, 2019
MRP: ₹425/-

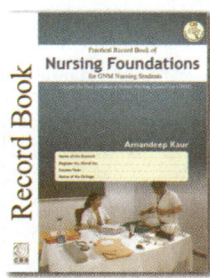
ISBN: 978-93-88178-50-1
Pages: 166   1/e, 2018-19
MRP: ₹350/-

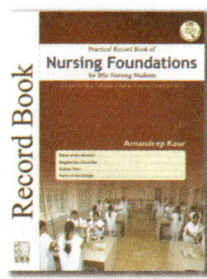
ISBN: 978-93-88108-96-6
Pages: 256   1/e, 2018-19
MRP: ₹425/-

Pharmacology/MSN

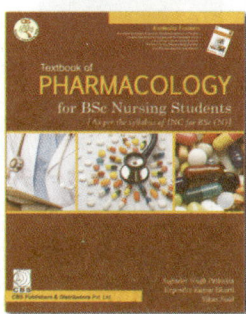
ISBN: 978-93-86217-80-6
Pages: 486   1/e, 2017-18
MRP: ₹625/-

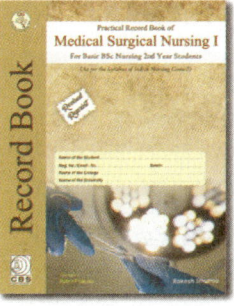
ISBN: 978-81-23928-00-5
Pages: 528   1/e, 2018-19
MRP: ₹550/-

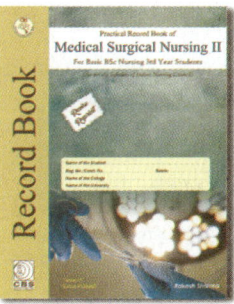
ISBN: 978-81-23928-01-2
Pages: 324   1/e, 2018-19
MRP: ₹475/-

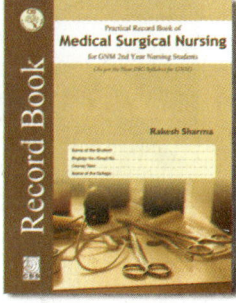
ISBN: 978-93-86827-04-3
Pages: 394   1/e, 2017
MRP: ₹475/-

Read, Review & Buy

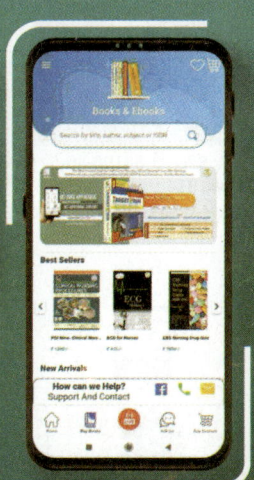

y, buying CBS Nursing Books is extra
convenient with Nursing Next Live Mobile App.

Glimpse of **Sample Pages and TOC** before you proceed to buy books.

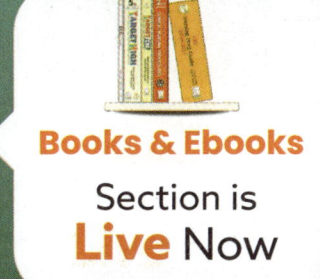

Books & Ebooks
Section is **Live** Now

Best Discounts &
Special Offers on all
the Books.

Child Health Nursing/Mental Health Nursing

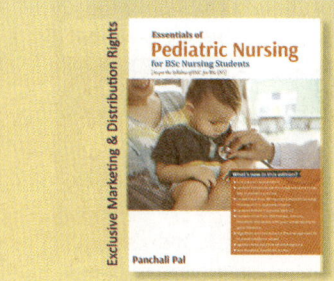

Exclusive Marketing & Distribution Rights

ISBN: 978-81-948693-2-0
Pages: 584   2/e, 2021
MRP: ₹795/-

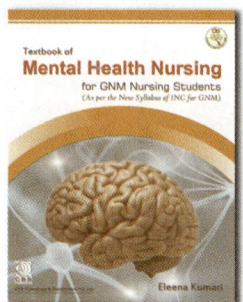

ISBN: 978-93-86827-48-7
Pages: 290   1/e, 2018
MRP: ₹310/-

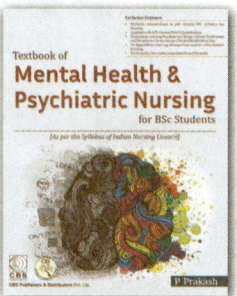

ISBN: 978-93-89261-91-2
Pages: 500   1/e, 2019
MRP: ₹625/-

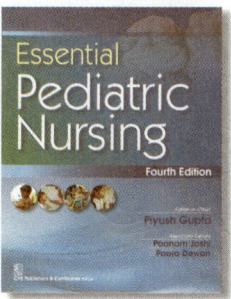

ISBN: 978-93-86217-87-5
Pages: 576   4/e, 2017
MRP: ₹750/-

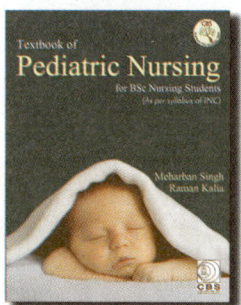

ISBN: 978-93-88108-72-0
Pages: 630   1/e, 2018
MRP: ₹725/-

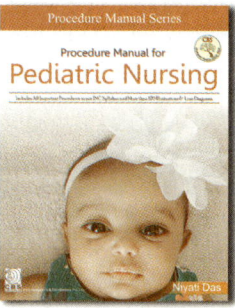

ISBN: 978-93-88108-86-7
Pages: 235   1/e, 2018
MRP: ₹325/-

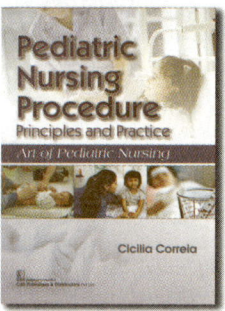

ISBN: 978-93-86310-74-3
Pages: 360   1/e, 2017
MRP: ₹450/-

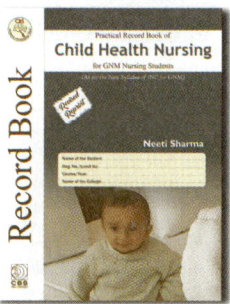

ISBN: 978-93-86827-53-1
Pages: 156   1/e, 2019
MRP: ₹325/-

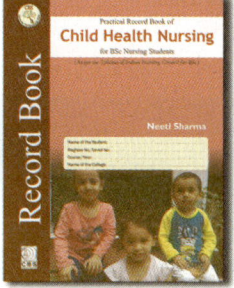

ISBN: 978-93-86827-05-0
Pages: 160   1/e, 2017
MRP: ₹310/-

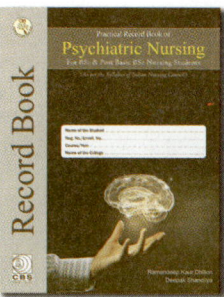

ISBN: 978-93-88108-80-5
Pages: 334   1/e, 2019
MRP: ₹415/-

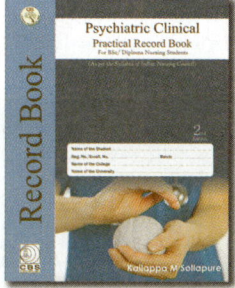

ISBN: 978-93-88108-81-2
Pages: 230   2/e, 2018-19
MRP: ₹395/-

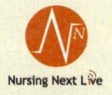

Midwifery, Obstetrical and Gynecological Nursing

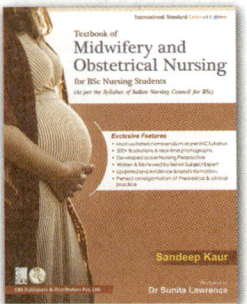

ISBN: 978-93-89261-90-5
Pages: 784   1/e, 2020
MRP: ₹995

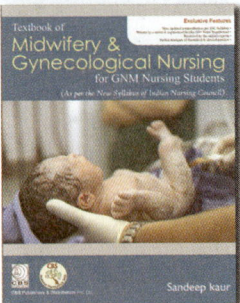

ISBN: 978-93-88108-83-6
Pages: 640   1/e, 2018
MRP: ₹625/-

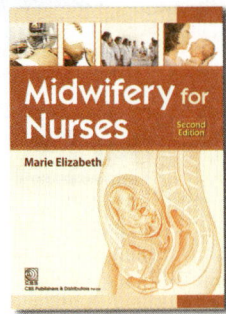

ISBN: 978-81-23922-14-0
Pages: 544   2/e, 2018
MRP: ₹650/-

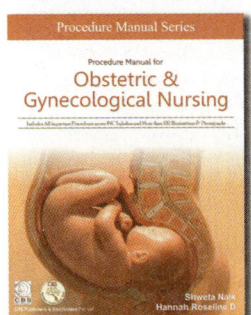

ISBN: 978-93-88178-60-0
Pages: 200   1/e, 2018-19
MRP: ₹235/-

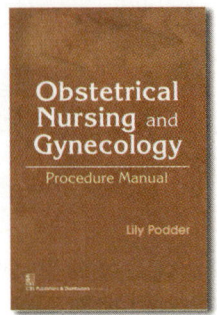

ISBN: 978-81-23925-81-3
Pages: 116   1/e, 2017
MRP: ₹265/-

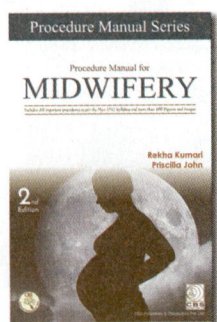

ISBN: 978-93-89261-94-3
Pages: 200   2/e, 2019
MRP: ₹225/-

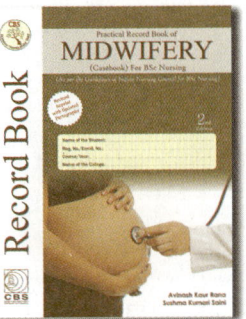

ISBN: 978-93-88178-65-5
Pages: 634 2/e (R/R), 2018-19
MRP: ₹675/-

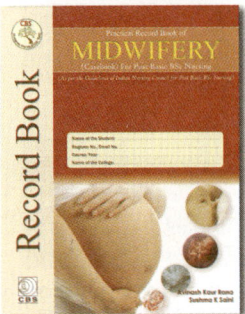

ISBN: 978-81-23927-07-7
Pages: 570   1/e, 2017
MRP: ₹375/-

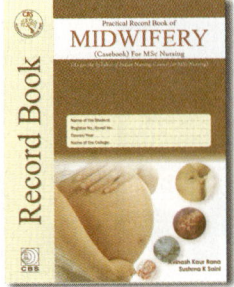

ISBN: 978-93-86217-97-4
Pages: 464   1/e, 2017
MRP: ₹625/-

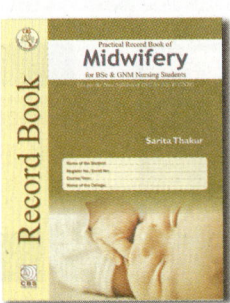

ISBN: 978-93-86827-33-3
Pages: 350   1/e, 2020
MRP: ₹415/-

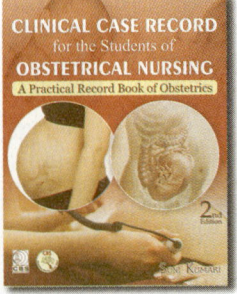

ISBN: 978-93-88178-51-8
Pages: 452   2/e, 2018
MRP: ₹475/-

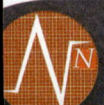
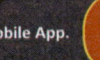
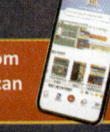

Nursing Research & Statistics/Management of Nursing Services & Education

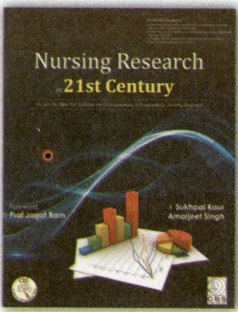

ISBN: 978-93-89261-89-9
Pages: 700   1/e, 2020
MRP: ₹725/-

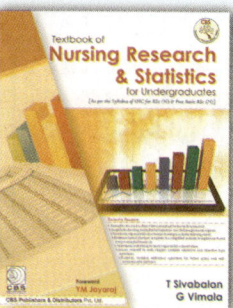

ISBN: 978-93-88178-61-7
Pages: 290   1/e, 2018
MRP: ₹525/-

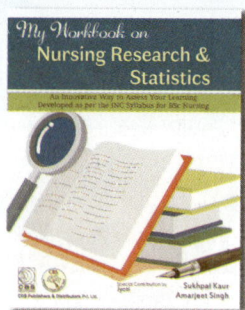

ISBN: 978-93-88108-75-1
Pages: 80   1/e, 2019
MRP: ₹150/-

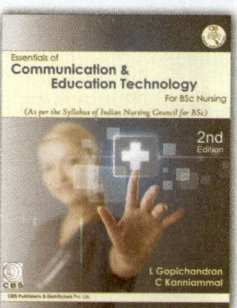

ISBN: 978-93-88178-58-7
Pages: 325   2/e, 2019
MRP: ₹475/-

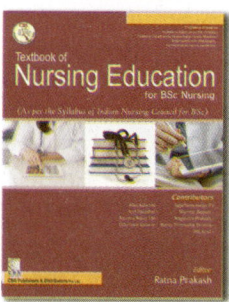

ISBN: 978-93-86827-34-0
Pages: 340   1/e, 2018
MRP: ₹450/-

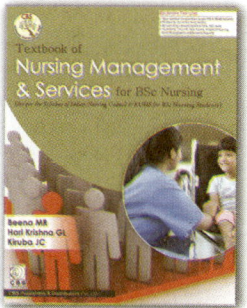

ISBN: 978-93-88178-62-4
Pages: 240   1/e, 2019
MRP: ₹625/-

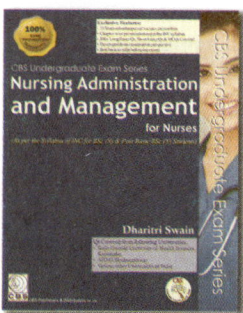

ISBN: 978-93-86827-42-5
Pages: 345   1/e, 2018
MRP: ₹350/-

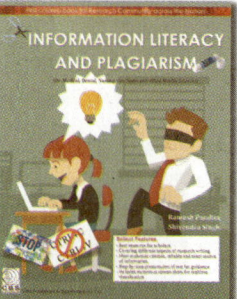

ISBN: 978-93-86827-13-5
Pages: 200   1/e, 2018
MRP: ₹370/-

Microbiology

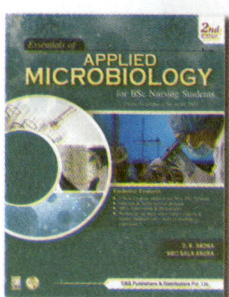

ISBN: 978-81-945234-4-4
Pages: 360   2/e, 2020-21
MRP: ₹575/-

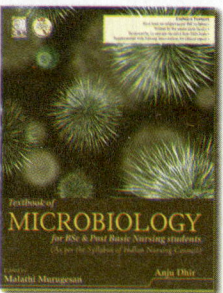

ISBN: 978-93-88108-82-9
Pages: 568   2/e, 2018
MRP: ₹725/-

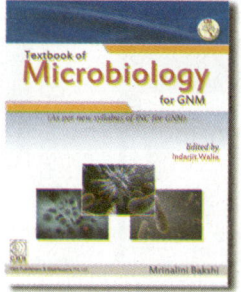

ISBN: 978-93-86827-23-4
Pages: 130   1/e, 2018
MRP: ₹225/-

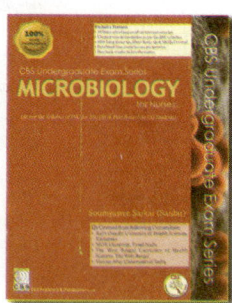

ISBN: 978-93-86310-49-1
Pages: 270   1/e, 2017
MRP: ₹275/-

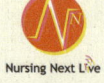

Anatomy & Physiology / Biochemistry & Nutrition/Sociology/Psychology

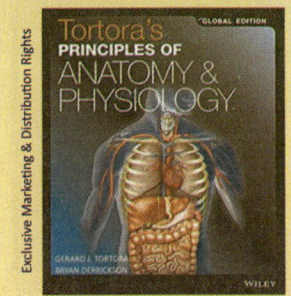

ISBN 978-81-26567614
Pages 1288   2/e, 2018
MRP: ₹3495/-

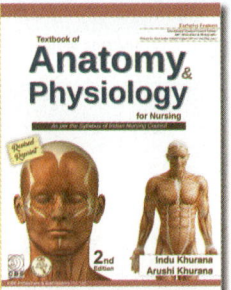

ISBN: 978-93-86827-12-8
Pages: 568   2/e, 2018
MRP: ₹995/-

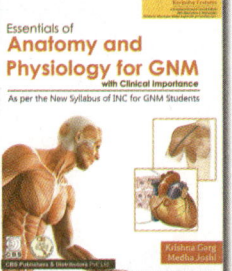

ISBN: 978-93-86827-11-1
Pages: 312   1/e, 2018
MRP: ₹475/-

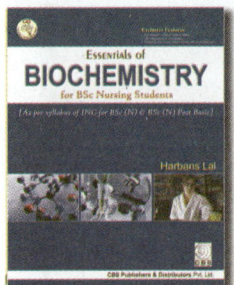

ISBN: 978-81-23927-19-0
Pages: 332 1/e (R/R), 2020-21
MRP: ₹450/-

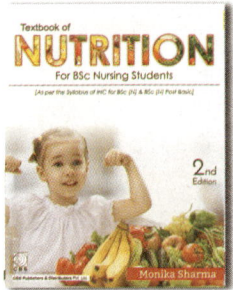

ISBN: 978-93-89261-92-9
Pages: 330   2/e, 2019
MRP: ₹370/-

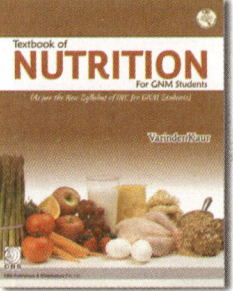

ISBN: 978-93-86827-10-4
Pages: 175   1/e, 2018
MRP: ₹275/-

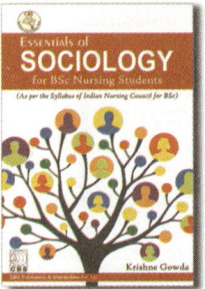

ISBN: 978-93-86217-51-6
Pages: 362   1/e, 2017
MRP: ₹395/-

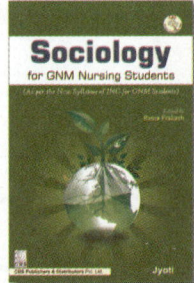

ISBN: 978-93-86827-26-5
Pages: 168   1/e, 2018
MRP: ₹210/-

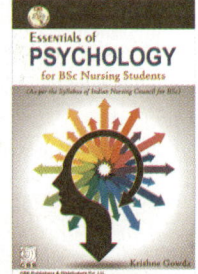

ISBN: 978-81-23927-11-4
Pages: 362   1/e, 2017
MRP: ₹340/-

English/First Aid/ Computer

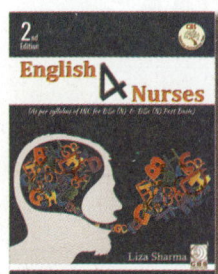

ISBN: 978-93-89261-95-0
Pages: 460   2/e, 2019
MRP: ₹415/-

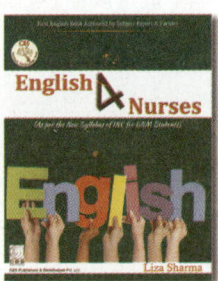

ISBN: 978-93-86827-09-8
Pages: 382   1/e, 2017
MRP: ₹350/-

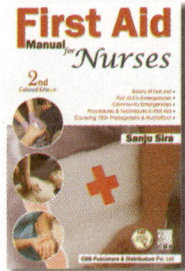

ISBN: 978-93-88178-55-6
Pages: 212   2/e, 2019
MRP: ₹310/-

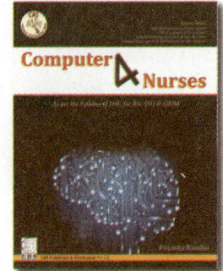

ISBN: 978-93-86310-48-4
Pages: 256   1/e, 2017
MRP: ₹370/-

Read, Review & Buy

Now, buying CBS Nursing Books is extra convenient with **Nursing Next Live** Mobile App.
Get a Glimpse of Sample Pages and TOC before you proceed to buy book.

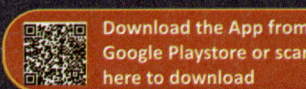

Download the App from Google Playstore or scan here to download

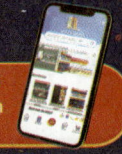

Others

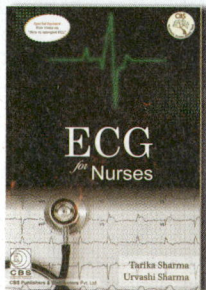

ISBN: 978-93-89261-88-2
Pages: 190   1/e, 2019
MRP: ₹415/-

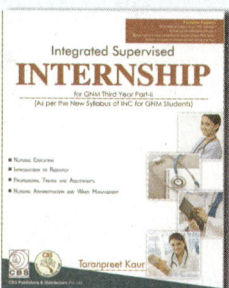

ISBN: 978-93-88108-89-8
Pages: 265   1/e, 2018
MRP: ₹415/-

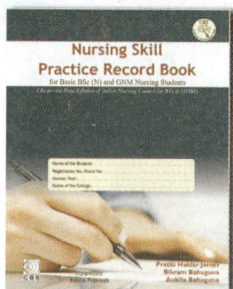

ISBN: 978-93-86827-38-8
Pages: 232   1/e, 2018-19
MRP: ₹310/-

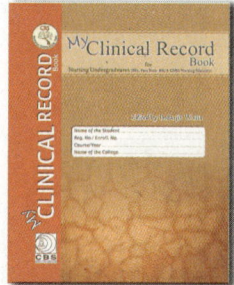

ISBN: 978-81-23927-04-6
Pages: 300   1/e, 2017-18
MRP: ₹325/-

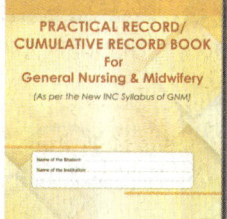

ISBN: 978-93-86827-03-6
Pages: 64   1/e, 2018
MRP: ₹225/-

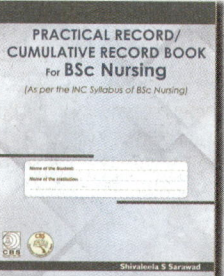

ISBN: 978-93-86827-01-2
Pages: 80   1/e, 2017
MRP: ₹210/-

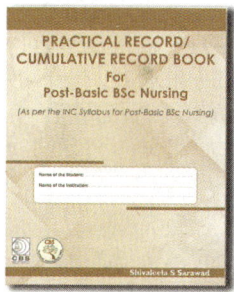

ISBN: 978-93-86827-02-9
Pages: 48   1/e, 2018
MRP: ₹225/-

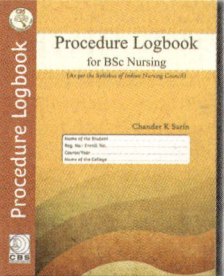

ISBN: 978-93-86310-46-0
Pages: 80   1/e, 2017
MRP: ₹210/-

Nursing Next Live

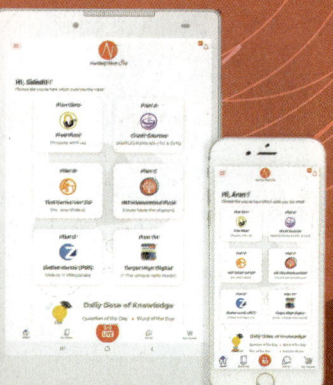

The Complete Package

- 40,000+ MCQs with Rationale
- 2000+ Hours of Recorded video lectures (Covering All Subjects/All Topics /Imp Topics Chanting Videos/Exam Discussions/LMR/IBQ & VBQs Discussions)
- 150+ Previous years' question papers covering all National & State Level Exams (2020-10)
- Monthly Live Doubt Sessions
- 200+ Newly Created Subject-wise cum Topic-wise Test, Mini Test & Grand Tests based on all important National Exams like AIIMS, PGIMER, JIPMER, DSSSB, RRB & ESIC, also State level exams like Kerala PSC
- 1500+ E-Notes/Flash cards of all the subjects for Last-Minute Revision
- 1000+ Image-based Questions with Rationale
- 200+ Video-based Questions with Rationale
- Monthly National Scholarship Test with Reward points
- 200+ CBS Nursing Books available for purchase

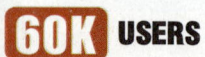 **60K** USERS

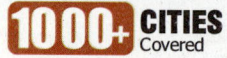 **1000+** CITIES Covered

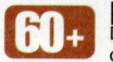 **60+** Mins Daily Average Time of users

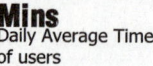

 **4.7** ★ RATINGS Google Play Store